WHAT

Divya Jyoti h
teach. Like a .... child, it gives me immense
joy seeing her grow and evolve much farther than her
own expectations. She is not only living the teachings,
she is also helping others to learn, grow and progress
spiritually. She is carrying on the teacher/disciple lineage
of Sri Sivananda and passing on the yogic spiritual
philosophy to her own students. This little book on
Living Yoga will help those who really want to know
what yoga is all about. It will help them transform and
evolve.

I am happy that Divya has made the yogic philosophy
her own and has become one with it. My loving blessings
to her and to all her students on the spiritual path.

Om!!
Swamini Lalitanda Saraswati Mataji
President
Atma Vidya Ashram

The personal experiences of the author, Divya Jyoti, and
her clear understanding and teaching of the philosophy
of living yoga in daily life will resonate not only with the
novice, but with people who have been living yoga for
many years. Divya Jyoti's simple way of explaining truth
is enlightening and powerful and has personally helped
me to reassess how I can stay on the path with strength
and determination. Divya reminds us that we are all
pearls on string with no separation from each other or
God and that everything we do has a direct effect on
everyone else.

Deborah Tostanowski
Boynton Beach, Fl.

"Living Yoga" gives practical insight into the practice of yoga in daily life. It is very helpful and inspiring for spiritual seekers all over the world. The value of the book is further enhanced by the fact that it is to raise funds in the USA for the Atma Vidya Ashram for it's humanitarian activities.

You have my blessings and prayers that your book may waft the aroma of Satyam-Shivam-Sundaram (Truth-Auspiciousness-Beauty) in the heart of spiritual seekers all over the world!

May God bless you, Swamini Lalitananda, and all those who are dedicated to charitable activities.

> With regards Prem and Om,
> Yours in the Lord,
> Swami Jyotirmayananda
> Yoga Research Foundation
> So. Miami, FL

Warning! This short and easily read book is deceptive in its simplicity! It's full of power and the glory of the divine! In sharing the ways in which she herself has applied the universal and basic tenets of yoga to her everydayreal Americanlife—a life to which anyone can relate—Patty (Divya Jyoti) DiFazio pulls the curtain back on deep spiritual matters and breaks it down into bite-sized, digestible spiritual food. If you have ever wondered what it is like to be a mystic in ordinary clothing, this combination of memoir and teachings will let you in on the experience. And if you have ever wondered HOW to become a mystic in ordinary clothing, this book is for you! Delve into the richness of yoga applied to your life beyond the physical practices most associate with the term. Patty DiFazio is a true "yogini"; take this walk with her through *Living Yoga*.

> *Rev. Nettie M. Spiwack*
> *www.nettiespiwack.com*

I started reading your book a couple of days ago. Tears have been pouring, not for sadness, but for joy. Only a devotee could have had such experiences as you had. Your autobiography on the background and explanation of what you went through on your spiritual journey is amazing, uplifting and most astonishing. Rivers of ink have been used to explain Hinduism, Vedanta and yoga, it's teachings, use and applications by unnumbered scholars and pundits. Patty, you've outdone them all with the simplicity of your heart and love. In a simple and concise way, you'd make anyone that reads your book understand the message and put those teachings into daily practice.

Antonio LoGrasso
Savannah, GA

"Living Yoga" by Patricia DiFazio is written in a lovely conversational style with personal stories which help illustrate the information presented on yoga philosophy, in a very simple, informative and accessible way. Divya takes us on her journey from the chapter on "Baby Steps" all the way through to "Look Within" with the message to embody your yoga...and she certainly does. "Go within and you shall find."

Paula Scopino LMT, E_RYT500, IAYT
Owner/Director Sacred Rivers Yoga Studio
Glastonbury, CT.

Congratulations on your wonderful book. I am sure it will be a great inspiration to those seeking the truth. I wish you success with your book and your path.
Many blessings from Yogi Hari.

Om Shanti,,Tara,
Yogi Hari's Ashram
Miramar, FL

Please send me ten copies of your book "Living Yoga." I want to give it free to my next set of classes in June. It was a read so easy and inviting and real and useful and inspiring to me that I want to pass it on.

Nicholaes Roosevelt
Yoga Instructor
UConn
Storrs, CT

I was expecting a book with all different yoga exercises, as I associate you with them from all these years of attending the retreat. But what a fantastic surprise! I was reading it in my back yard, I felt as if you were sitting in front of me and relating to me all those events. I could hear your voice and felt the warmth in my heart."

Dr. Indra Mohindra
Boston, MA

With Blessings from
Poojya Swamiji Dayananda Saraswathi

Best Wishes from
Sri Swamiji Tathvavidananda Saraswathi

Living Yoga

*Personal experiences
in applying
the philosophy of yoga
in daily life*

Patricia (Divya Jyoti) DiFazio

Library of Congress Catalog Number:
ISBN: 978-0-578-10545-1

Published by Living Yoga Books
All artwork by Patricia DiFazio
Book design and layout by Jonathan Gullery

Printed in Bangalore, India.

Printed by:
CYNOSURE MEDIA SOLUTIONS
#66, 4th Main, 1st Stage, 1st Phase, Manjunathnagar,
BANGALORE - 560010, Karnataka, India.
Ph: +91 80 2338 6271, Mob: +91 94481 74261
Email: cynosuremediasolutions@gmail.com

www.livingyogabooks.com

CONTENTS

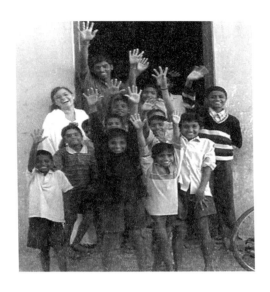

Profits from the sale of this book goes to support the Atma Vidya Ashram, which is a volunteer-based organization. Administrative expenses are very low. As a result, your contribution is utilized for helping the needy and most disadvantaged in India by providing food, clothing, medical care, and education at five orphanages and an old age home.

For further information and if you'd like to
Sponsor children, please visit:
www.Atma-Vidya.org

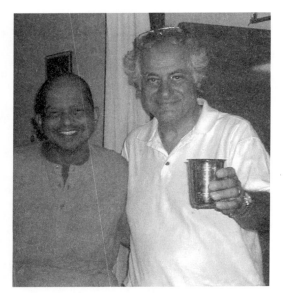

Omananda and Chuck

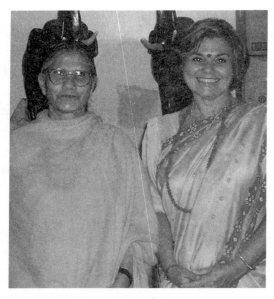

Swamiji and Divya

Dedication

I dedicate this book to the children of India
supported by the
Atma Vidya Ashram,

With gratitude, love and respect,

to
Swamini Lalitananda

and
to the memory of
Swami Omananda

and to the dedicated volunteers who have spent
countless hours caring for and raising funds for
this noble cause.

ACKNOWLEDGEMENT

I WOULD like to thank my husband Chuck DiFazio for being such a patient and loving partner on this journey. Without you, Chuck, I would not have traveled to India nor sat in the presence of Sri Sathya Sai Baba. Without you Chuck, I would not have had the confidence to venture into the unknown regions of my deepest self, to find my self. Without your selfless love, I would not have been able to open our home and heart to Swamini Lalitananda and the helpless children and elderly souls in India.

It is with deep love that I acknowledge you as a great man, and my soul mate on this journey.

I would like to thank my spiritual grand-daughter, Mariah (Prema Jyoti) for inspiration and technical support in the preparation of this book. To the jnani sisterhood, especially Mala and Nadine, for their love and encouragement. To my yoga students, I am grateful for the opportunity to teach what I love. To all of my children: Marc, Andy, Leslie, Andrea, Garrett and their spouses, thank you, I couldn't have done it without you. To Durga, Chuck, and Erin for your editing and encouragement. To my grandchildren, Lyndsey, Aimee, Monica, Felicia, Nicholas, Anya, Lukas, Griffin and

Ryan, this book is to help you remember your Nonnie and how much I love you. To my parents, I must have done something very good in a prior life to have gotten such wonderful parents. You inspire me to be the best that I can be.

If I have left your name out, please know that I acknowledge you as my own self and love you unconditionally.

I acknowledge my spiritual teachers: Sri Sathya Sai Baba, Swamini Lalitananda, Rajam Kumar, Swami Dayananda, Swami Jyothirmayananada, Yogi Hari, Yogi Amrit DeSai, Yogi Bhajan, Mother Meera, Mata Amritanandamayi, Shree Ma and the many beautiful souls that have touched my soul through yoga classes and spiritual discourses.

Through this book, I hope to illustrate how to weave the knowledge gained from these great teachers into daily life.

INTRODUCTION

WELCOME to Living Yoga.

The idea to write this book came as an extension of an outline for a Yoga Teacher Training program that I teach at the Sacred Rivers Yoga Studio in Glastonbury, CT.

I felt that students might like to read a little bit about my life as a living yogi, prior to taking my class in yogic philosophy. I e-mailed the outline to the students who were scheduled for the training, with the hope that if they read it, we would have a more interactive class.

The response to the class was very positive, and the outline began to get filled out with more stories and anecdotes from my life. What started as an explanation of the great sage Patanjali and how he organized the eight limbs of yoga, became the story of how an average American woman with a family became a spiritual seeker and a practicing yogini.

My quest for a fulfilling spiritual path brought me to India ten times and to the feet of some of the greatest spiritual teachers of this age. Taking this knowledge and the experiences that it afforded me and bringing them back into daily life, is what I hope this book conveys. Living Yoga is more than the regular practice of yoga postures. Living yoga is the practice of yoga in daily life. How can we practice yoga in daily life without "doing" yoga?' you may ask. "Don't do: BE" is the response my teacher would give. <u>Be a yogi or yogini by living the teachings of the great philosophy of yoga.</u> This little book will help you to understand how to BE a yogi. Many words used in this book are in the Sanskrit language. I translate each word, but have also included a glossary in the back for you to refer to.

I truly hope that you enjoy this book and the journey that you are about to begin. It is now time to get off your yoga mat and get into the life that you have only imagined existed. I promise you that following a yogic life-style will lead you to your deeper self, your authentic self, and that is a path worth following.

Namaste',
Patty (Divya Jyoti) DiFazio

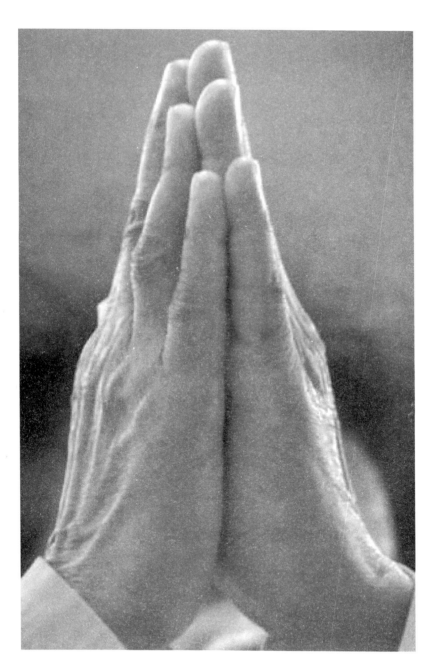

LEARNING TO WALK

SISTER Veronica looked out over the heads of the children as she drilled them with questions from the Baltimore Catechism. We had all studied the questions in fear that when the Bishop quizzed us, we might not answer correctly. "Oh no" I thought, "if I answer the question wrong, I'll get a big black mark on my soul." Sister Veronica tapped her starched pure white bib and assured us that our innocent souls were as white as her bib.

"Where is God?" she asked. "God is everywhere," we responded in unison. Then my mind would go off thinking about that profound question. "If God is everywhere, why can't we see him everywhere?"

"God lives in our heart" the children responded to the question I'd missed in my musings.

"Oh, that's right," I thought. That's how HE can be everywhere; He's in ALL of our hearts." So every day I would talk to God in my heart.

"Please bless Aunt Joyce and the new baby that

is coming soon," I'd pray. I was diligent about praying for babies because I wasn't sure that they would all make it into the earth plane without a lot of direction. With lots of brothers, sisters and cousins surrounding me, I led the pack like the Pied Piper, pretty certain that God really did listen to me. But who was I that God would listen to me?

Even at this young age, I would stand on a step stool and stare into my eyes in the bathroom mirror. I'd mentally ask God "But who am I really? Who is in there watching me, watch me? Is it You, God?" I asked. Little did I know that those questions of introspection were deeply philosophical.

At age eight, I was a young blossoming yogi. Of course I didn't even know the word yogi at that time, but I was always a spiritually inquisitive child. At recess time at school, while the other children were playing group sports or climbing on the monkey bars, I would be playing in the fields nearby, imagining that I was a nun in a convent. I even thought about joining a convent, but that didn't seem right either. I loved family and children too much to live in solitude.

"But where did I come from?" I asked as I stared into my mirror. Now there's a deep question for an eight year old. Maybe I knew, deep down, that I had lived before and was born this time to experience the answers to these questions by *living yoga*.

What in the world is *living yoga*?

Living yoga is a phrase that I coined to describe the lifestyle of a yogi who lives his/her yoga every day. But it wasn't for another twenty years that I would experience yoga.

Most people in the United States think of yoga as some kind of physical fitness program where we get into pretzel like postures and make funny sounds. As a matter of fact, the first time I did yoga with my mother, back in the 1970's, we left the yoga class laughing at the funny chanting going on. What I didn't realize until later, much later, was that the laughter that we just couldn't stop, was a euphoric feeling that came from the energy gained from deep breathing and the chanting that we did that night. I also had no idea that a yoga class in the basement of a church in Old Saybrook, CT would change my life. I would continue to do yoga for the next 30 plus years and continue to practice it to this very day.

MEETING MY LIFE'S PARTNER

"YOU will meet her through your work", Aida said. "I want to say, across your desk."

Chuck often visited his seventy-eight year old friend Aida, a gifted psychic who was able to tune into him dramatically. A few weeks later, Aida called Chuck and announced: "You've met the woman I was telling you about," and went on to describe me, in detail, to my future husband. The story of our romance is very sweet. Aida told us that we had lived together in previous lives and had to help each other grow spiritually in this life much like Ruth and Boaz in the Story of Ruth in the Old Testament. In fact, when we married, we incorporated the "Song of Ruth" into the wedding service:

Wherever you go, I will go
Wherever you live, so shall I live
Your people will be my people
And your God will be my God too.

Little did we know how right Aida's prediction was. Together, over time, we would adopt a new set of spiritual principles and follow a different spiritual path.

After that first night of yoga, with my mother many years ago, I continued to do yoga and my life went on as usual. I had a career and two children when I fell in love with Chuck. Together we pursued our dreams that took us from a traditional life in a house overlooking the Connecticut River, to Prasanthi Nilayam (the Abode of Peace), Sathya Sai Baba's ashram in India. Chuck's attraction to this spiritual teacher gave my life a whole new dimension. I started reading and following his teachings. I began to practice Baba's "human values" of love, non-violence, truth, peace, and right action. Many years, and several trips to India, living in the ashram and practicing yoga on rooftops, passed by before I connected the teachings of Jesus Christ and Sathya Sai Baba to the teachings of the great sage Patanjali.

"Boy, these aren't so different from Baba's teachings," I thought. Baba had been drumming these principles into my head for 20 years, and the Catholic nuns before that. In order to pass my yoga teacher training test, I studied the yogic principles of Patanjali that are necessary to control our senses. These principles are called "Yamas," and they mirror the teachings of Sathya Sai Baba and many of the great saints and teachers of all religions. I share them with you now, because I feel that they really help us to move forward and understand what "Living Yoga" means.

BEYOND THE VEIL

AIDA was the first psychic I had ever met and it scared me a little to think that someone could go into a meditative state and be able to connect so fully that she knew everything about me, in this lifetime and in others. But soon, I too began having deeply meaningful psychic experiences.

Not long after our marriage, my Great Aunt Pauline, who had passed on, appeared to me in my bedroom. She looked exactly as I remembered her in life, rocking to and fro in her rocking chair and smiling at me.

"Chuck, Aunt Paul's here," I whispered as I shook my husband's shoulder.

"What?" he asked bleary eyed.

"Aunt Paul. She's here, in the room...up by the ceiling"

"That's nice," mumbled my sleepy spouse. "What does she want?"

"Nothing. She's not saying anything, but she's smiling. I think she's happy that we "found each other."

"Me too," he said as he drifted back to sleep.

Several times after that, Aunt Paul would appear, like the Cheshire cat, smiling and rocking in her chair, just looking over us and blessing us from beyond.

My Uncle Nick is another soul who found me to be

an open channel for communication. My father's brother had died of cancer leaving a wife and young family of six children. I had been the flower girl in their wedding and as their family grew, baby sitter for all of their children. Uncle Nick worked all his life with my Dad in their store. We were a very close family. Summers were spent near the ocean, in a cluster of summer cottages. It was a little family compound of uncles, aunts and dozens of cousins.

One morning, I went out in the yard at the beach to tell my Aunt that Uncle Nick had visited me. She smiled and asked if he had a message for her. I told her that he just wanted her to know that he loved her. She started to cry and said;

"Today is our wedding anniversary."

An open channel you ask? How can we open up and connect to something that is beyond the veil? In my case, these 'appearances' happened spontaneously. I wasn't soliciting a response from any disembodied spirit, and I began to question it myself. Is this my mind making stuff up? Are there really other dimensions with other beings that we cannot see? It seemed that these 'communications' came when I was totally relaxed.

"Maybe it's connected to meditation in some way" I thought. Sathya Sai Baba seems to know every thought in my mind. He even responds to my thoughts without me even verbalizing them. Mother Meera is another amazing saint in whose presence, I experience deep levels of awareness. When she looked into my eyes, I fell into such a deep reverie, colors spun around my head. Thus, meditation became another step for me along the yogic path.

People often ask me "Do you do yoga and meditate every day?" At age 66 I may not practice yoga postures every day but I *live* yoga every day and that's what I'd like to share with you.

YAMAS–ABSTENTIONS
THE DON'T'S

1. AHIMSA- DO NO HARM – (NON-VIOLENCE)

YES! That human value number one is there in Sai Baba's teachings as well as in the message of most religious philosophies like the Ten Commandments' directive, "Thou shalt not kill!"

At its deepest level, *ahimsa* non-violence, means that we need to keep from harming any living thing, starting with ourselves. This concept of not harming usually translates in our mind as no physical violence. I describe this as "oh, I would never hurt anybody," but what about harsh and hurtful words? Words are weapons as harmful as knives but can cut even deeper. This is the very first principle. Watch our words. Watch our thoughts. Thoughts can harm us from within making us angry or aggressive. Watch our actions. Do not strike out at others. Non-violence means not harming anyone in thoughts, words or actions.

Are we kind and gentle with ourselves? Or are we "people pleasers" doing what others want and never really caring for ourselves. "Do no harm" means to take care of our precious bodies and minds. We cannot even begin to recognize the God within if we don't honor our body as the temple of God.

Do no harm to any living being, translates to:

"Don't kill living beings for pleasure."

At some point in the practice of yoga, you will probably come to the realization that eating the flesh of animals is wrong. In our culture we package it at the supermarket to keep from relating to the fact that it is a dead animal.

When I was six years old, I used to walk from my dad's market up the hill to our home. On the way, I passed the chicken market. The back room had a large plate glass window that I would peer into to see the chickens in their coops. One day, just as I walked by, whap! The chicken's head fell to the floor. I was horrified, and from that day on, I'd walk by that window with my hand up like a blinder to keep from witnessing that scene again.

One day, my Dad asked me why I never wave to Uncle Joe in the chicken market any more. I had some explaining to do.

It was many years later, when Chuck and I had adopted a vegetarian lifestyle, that I was finally able to explain to my father how killing animals, chicken or fish was a violent act and that eating the bodies of these once living beings, was no longer possible for me. Having owned a market that sold fresh meats and then a family-run seafood restaurant, Dad never held the same views, but he accepted me and my lifestyle of adhering to *ahimsa*.

2. SATHYAM- TRUTH

This human value is also one we have been taught by our parents, schoolteachers, and religious mentors. However,falsehood has become a way of life for many people. Truth can be relative for humans. I strive to be truthful unless that truth would be harmful to others. My truth may not be your truth. They say that beauty is in the eye of the beholder. Giving compliments, just to make someone feel good, is not necessarily "truth." Speaking about people behind their back, gossiping, engaging in mindless chatter are all ways of bending the truth and better left unsaid. How much time do you spend on the telephone, cell phone, texting or e-mailing. Is it true? Is it necessary?

Take a good look at what motivates you to say the things you say and try to speak the truth, to the best of your ability. This is not easy, but a worthwhile challenge.

Sai Baba teaches that the deepest truth is that which never changes. Now that is something to ponder. As we move through these pages, that concept will begin to get clearer.

3. ASTEYA-NON-STEALING

Wow, this is beginning to sound like the Ten Commandments. Didn't Moses have that written on his tablet of stone? Thousands of years before Moses, asteya was a moral concept in the Far East, meaning more than just not taking material things from others. It means not taking away someone's self-respect or confidence. We hear a great deal about bullying in schools, razing in college or the military, disparaging comments about gays, pediphilia and rape. These actions take away self esteem creating a worthlessness in people. Don't steal anything from another.

Asteya also means not stealing ideas and giving credit where credit is due.

I should probably be listing not only all of my amazing teachers, but every book, article or lecture I've ever heard in the credits for this book. NONE of the concepts that I write about here, except for personal experiences, are original to me. All have been passed down from the great sages, swamis and yogis of old. I honor them all and give all credit to them for the words that you are reading now. This is the practice of *asteya*.

4. APARIGRAHA– FREEDOM FROM ATTACHMENT. NON-COVETNESSNESS

Now, where did I hear that before? Greed is so prevalent in our society. We always seem to strive for a bigger house, nicer car or a better paying job. I have known some pretty wealthy people who seem to identify with their money. "I am rich," becomes who they are. Then there are those who like to brag about their children and the Ivy League college that they got into or the pride they have that their son is a doctor. This is attachment. Unfortunately, these individuals are in for a huge disappointment if they lose their money or if their offspring turn out to be a disappointment. I had an Indian woman in one of my yoga classes who was distraught about her son. Many years ago,this adult son had brought a young woman home to meet his parents, but mom did not approve of his choice and refused to allow her son to marry. The son is still single, and the woman has no grandchildren. She blames herself for her son's unhappiness, and cries for her own loneliness. This striving for control over another person is attachment. At some point every parent needs to detach from their children, knowing that karma will play out with or without their personal direction.

Thou shalt not covet thy neighbor's goods. Why not? Because having your neighbor's possessions will not bring you true joy. To want and or revel in that which is not yours, is coveting. I've heard of people who won the lottery and after years of mismanagement, died penniless. There are also stories of people who frequent casinos. Even the big winners end up losers.I think that maybe by taking that which belonged to another, they also took on their *karma*. A yogi looks at desires versus needs, and does not covet what he does not need.

5. BRAMACHARAYA –SEXUAL CONTINENCE -SELF-CONTROL

In the case of a yogi, this refers to sexual purity. A yogi can be married, or in a committed relationship but should strive for chastity in thought, word, and deed. Desires and attachments are detrimental on the spiritual path. Although not required, many spiritual seekers choose to remain celibate and non-attached. That sexual energy that is not expelled can be diverted into spiritual energy for transformation.

In order to remember the eight limbs of yoga for my yoga teacher-training program, I drew a tree. And on

that tree, I put the five *yamas* as one of the thick roots
of the tree. If I can live the *yamas* and control my senses
as my foundation, I thought, then I am a living yogi. I've
had over twenty years of practicing the human values as
taught by my guru and fifty years of living by the Ten
Commandments as taught by my faith. I knew that I
could do this!

Then I looked at Patanjali's *niyamas* (considered
the second limb of yoga). Niyamas are those principles
needed to live a life of purity and for me, represent a
way of measuring my success on this path. These are the
results of practicing the five *yamas*.

NIYAMAS. OBSERVANCES: THE DO'S

1. TAPAS- AUSTERITY

SATHYA Sai Baba's "Ceiling on Desires" program helped me with this concept. He taught us to put a ceiling on our desires, to be generous and give away what we don't need and not acquire more than is necessary. At least once a year, Chuck and I clean out closets and drawers of clothing that we don't wear and donate it to St. Mary's Church.

Moderation is a good word to describe this *niyama*. Can we discipline ourselves? Can we set a schedule of work, pleasure,and spiritual study and stay in balance? A yogic lifestyle starts with a balanced lifestyle.

2. SHAUCHA-MENTAL AND PHYSICAL PURITY

If my mind/ body is the temple of God, then it is my duty to keep it pure and clean. There is no excuse for not bathing and wearing clean clothing. My environment also reflects this purity. My home is clean and unclut-tered in order to have a positive psychological effect upon me. I don't allow un-pure images to enter my mind via the computer, television, movies or newspapers. The foods I eat and the thoughts that I think must also be pure and loving.

3. SANTOSHA- CONTENTMENT

Living with my beloved husband helps to keep me content. I have all that I could want. Contentment is inner experience, versus happiness, which is often the result of an outside stimulus. Stop what you are engrossed in for a moment and reflect on how you are, in this moment. Are you content? In this moment, all is well. There is no past to worry about. The past is in the past. There is no future to worry about. The future has not yet arrived. In this moment, feel the peace of contentment. Occasionally, in the past, I would go visit our psychic friend Aida when life seemed overwhelming. Aida, in her very wise way, would look at me and say, "this too, shall pass," and you know what? It did.

4. SWADHYAYA-SELF-STUDY

For me, study is not only the study of scriptures, but also the repetition of *mantras* (a daily practice) and the daily reflection of how I am doing on my path of spiritual progress. For years, I used a journal as a way of tracking my meditations and experiences along this path. Some of those entries will appear further on in this book. More recently, I have started a study group of like-minded women to read and reflect. Everything we experience through our senses becomes a part of us.

I watch the things I see and hear, and like the three monkeys I see no evil, hear no evil and do no evil.

5. ISHWAR PRANIDHAN: SURRENDER TO GOD

Surrender does not mean to give up, but to entrust our lives to a higher power. We do the action, but realize that the universe itself is Divine Consciousness and we are a part of that Consciousness. When I intend to live in harmony with the Divine Consciousness, I realize unity with Divine Consciousness. Sai Baba said that we are like light bulbs with a current running through us. That current is the God energy. As we surrender to this energy, our light shines bright with no effort. It took years for me to truly understand the concept of surrendering to God. Part of that confusion was my image of who God was. The more I practiced a yogic lifestyle, the more I got away of the concept of god as a physical form and closer to understanding divinity as a cosmic Consciousness. I surrender to that.

I made the *niyamas* the second big fat root of my yogic tree, giving it stability and strength. Growing upward from this stable root system of *yamas and niyamas* (considered two of the limbs of yoga) grow the other six limbs of yoga as categorized by Patanjali.

As I continued my studies, I learned that in addition to the two roots, there are six more branches of yoga.

(1) ASANA: Postures

Asana are the physical postures that help strengthen

and steady our bodies. Moving our body into the various postures lubricates the joints and strengthens the muscles. Without a strong, flexible body, it is difficult to sit still in meditation. *Asana* also help us to prepare the body and energy channels for the movement of the divine energy or life force riding on the breath and called *prana*. *Asana* should not be done as a competitive sport. *Yoga* is not about competition or sculpting the perfect body. *Asana* is a step along the path, a branch on the tree leading to self-realization.

(2) PRANAYAMA: breath control (control of the life force within us)

How can we control our life force when we can't even control our thoughts? Actually, practicing the control of breathing helps us to watch our thoughts.

Prana, or divine life force, rides on the breath. This limb comes after *asana* to begin with a strong body able to hold this life force in the lungs and through the thousands of nadis (energy pathways in the physical body).

Through controlling the breath, we can have some control of this spiritual life force as it courses through the energetic pathways and *chakras* or energy vortexes.

(3) PRATYAHARA: sense control- the ability to not be distracted by the world

Our five senses are what bring us outside of ourselves and into the world. Our senses (sight, smell, touch, taste and hearing) make us aware of the beauty of the material world. However, our senses can turn us in a negative direction if we overdo or become attached to the material thing or idea that the senses direct us to. Learning how to control our desires that are stimulated by our senses is essential for spiritual progress. Sense control starts for me, by not listening to the radio, or watching TV. I don't need the over stimulation of the media to get my mind out into the world.

(4) DHARANA: concentration of the mind

Try being successful at anything (crossword puzzle, mathematics etc) without concentration. It's almost impossible. We must be able to focus the mind by shutting out the distractions that appear as thought waves or sense perceptions that distract us. There are many techniques to help us concentrate. Single pointed focus is essential.

(5) DHYANA: meditation

(moving from concentration, to contemplation to stillness)

Techniques to quiet the mind allow us to observe the thought waves without engaging them or acting on them This is meditation. There are many techniques to move into meditation. I suggest that you try them all until you find the one that works to still your thought waves, and then stick with it. The ability to quiet the thoughts to a steady, unwavering mind is meditation. Meditation is a permanent link to *Atma*, your link with divinity.

(6) SAMADHI: super consciousness
(Union with Divine Consciousness)

The interesting thing about this daunting goal, is that we are already there. Divinity is everywhere.

Picture deep, dark space as not empty, but Divine Consciousness itself. It has no form, no attributes at all, but it exists as consciousness everywhere. Anything that appears in that space is IN God. Planets,even whole galaxies emerge from within God. Forms appear as denser molecules.

As we move into the earth's atmosphere, gravity makes itself apparent. Humidity is a heaviness of water molecules and the denser it becomes, more form is evident until rain falls.

These raindrops exist within God, just as waves exist as forms that emerge out of the ocean.

There was a story told to me once about a huge wave that was very proud of his size and power. A smaller wave rolled along the surface of the sea more placidly. Soon, the huge wave realized that his destiny was landfall and he would very soon be crashing against the cliffs.

"Oh no," screamed the powerful wave. "I'll be smashed to smithereens. Aren't you scared?" he cried out to the little wave. And with a large crash and spray, the huge wave crashed into the cliff. The little wave rolled lazily up the rock surface and rolled back down gently merging with the sea.

All forms emerge from Divine Consciousness and merge back. Ego makes us think that we are separate from God.

The word *Atma* means the God within us. The word *Brahma* means the universal God. The eight limbs of yoga move us from our individual selves and *Atma* within to universal soul or *Brahma*. So, I travel from myself to my **self,** to realize **my Self.**

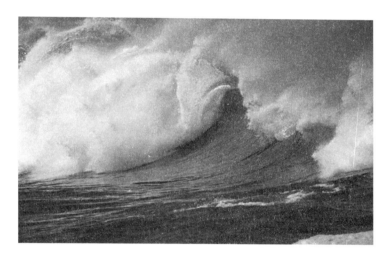

Think of it this way: When you start to create a document on your computer, you start with a blank screen. Form appears as words. If you are computer savvy, you may add another layer to your document in the form of a photo or graph. These forms appear on what was a blank screen. The screen is always there and the forms are layered upon it. Union with Divine Consciousness is a realization that God is always there, and we, as forms, are layered upon divinity. We are one and the same.

The ultimate goal of yoga, is this union with Divine Consciousness. As we get wrapped up following the path of yoga, we forget about the goal. That's a good thing.

With no attachment to the outcome, you will find that by following the path of these eight limbs of yoga, you will come to the realization that you have arrived. "Arrived where?" you ask. Right here, right now. You are **that**.

THE TREE OF YOGA

I DREW six branches of yoga as branches of my yogic tree. All together, the branches and roots of my tree show the eight limbs of yoga as described by the great sage Patanjali (Yamas and Niyamas as the root of the tree and six branches of the tree). I stress the importance of learning these eight limbs and practicing the Yamas and the Niyamas as the foundation of a yogic lifestyle. I find that most yoga classes in the United States, jump right into asana (yoga postures) without giving any credence to the spiritual structure of a yogic lifestyle at all. The yamas (abstentions) and the niyamas (observations) are often relegated to a secondary role if they are taught at all.

I feel that I was very lucky to have had the opportunity so early in life to sit at the feet of Sathya Sai Baba and learn how to live a spiritual life. My husband and I were both practicing these teachings when I came to know about the yoga aphorisms of Patanjali. Things began to click in my head. Baba's teachings are not unique to Him. Many other great masters taught the same concepts. They are laid out for us in the Upanishads of India. Patanjali compiled these teachings many years before the birth of Christ, even before Moses was given the Ten Commandments. I find it remarkable that

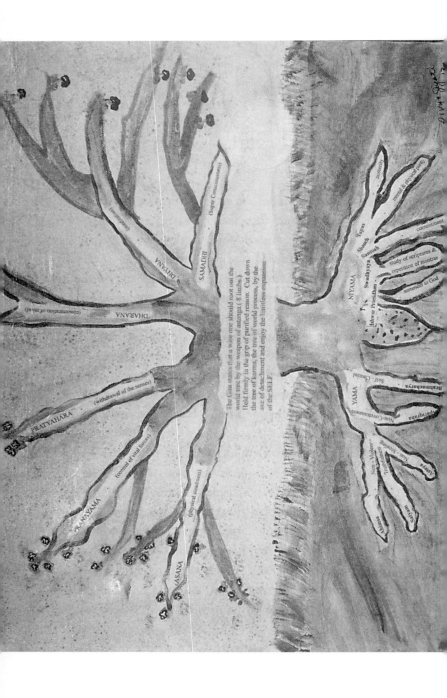

The Gita states that a wise one should root out the world tree by the weapon of asanga (8 limbs)
Held firmly in the grip of purified reason. Cut down the tree of karma, the tree or world process, by the axe of detachment and enjoy the limitless expansion of the SELF.

SAMADHI (Super Consciousness)

DHYANA (meditation)

DHARANA (concentration of mind)

PRATYAHARA (withdrawal of the senses)

PRANAYAMA (control of vital forces)

ASANA (physical steadiness)

NIYAMA

Zuiriry
mental & physical purity
contentment
study of scriptures & repetition of mantras
surrender to God

Tapas
Shauch
Santosh
Swadhyaya
Ishwar Pranidhan

YAMA

Self - Control
Non - Covetousness
Brahmacharya
Aprigrahas

Non - Stealing
Asteya
Non - Violence
Ahimsa
Truthfulness
Satya

the *yamas and niyamas* are so reminiscent of tablets of stone with rules or ethics handed to man from his God.

Look over my tree and trace the spiritual progress that leads from a strong foundation rooted in observances and abstentions...growing upward with the strength of postures and proper breathing, moving deeper with sense withdrawal, focus, concentration, and meditation. The goal of yoga is not only to grow a strong tree, but also to eventually, cut down the tree of *karma* and worldly passion with the ax of detachment, and enjoy the limitless expansion of the self. I hope to share this journey with you in the stories that follow.

Many years went by and I happily practiced yoga. At age 53, I retired from my career and became a full time yogi, teaching 8 classes a week. Yet, I wanted to know that I was still growing in awareness and making progress along the yogic path. I went back to the *Ashtanga* Eight Limbed path, my yogic tree, to revisit the *niyamas*. The real challenge of living a yogic lifestyle began. *Tapas* or "austerity" or "detachment" sounded scary. How could I be a wife and mother and detach from my family? I don't want to live as a swami. I love my life, my husband, children and my parents. Cut down the tree of worldly passion with the ax of detachment? I wasn't sure I was ready to do that. Then one day, about 15 years ago, I met a woman at the Hindu temple dressed in the orange sari of renunciation. We sat and talked until the temple was about to close. " Do you have a ride home?" I asked the swamini. "No, I'll just sleep here," she replied. I ended up bringing Swamini Lalitananda home with me and there she stayed. Swamiji, as I lovingly addressed her, taught me about detachment. Swamis renounce their former lives, like monks and nuns. They receive a new name and a new life serving the divine.

"How can I practice detachment as a householder?" I asked.

"Treat everyone as God" was her answer. "Nothing really belongs to you anyway. All things and all people are divine. Do your duty with no expectations."

Wow! O.K. here we go. I can't tell you that it was easy, but I can tell you that I did make an effort to live my life with no expectation or attachment to the outcome. This does not mean to stop loving family and friends; it means to not attach to how things may turn out. This was a challenge when family members faced drug addiction and cancer. But it helped, really it did, to not attach to an outcome. If the outcome were to be death, then I would face that when the time came. Cut down the tree of *karma* and worldly passion. What does that even mean? Let's take another look at that tree. Can you see all those seeds in the big thick taproot? Those seeds represent *karma*. *Karmas* are the results of our thoughts, words and deeds. These results must be balanced out. As long as we continue to create *karmas,* the tree continues to flower, and seed, and propagate. Detachment is the key. If we can manage to detach from the outcome or fruits of our actions, we pop the *karmic* seeds making it impossible for them to germinate. Be pure witness consciousness. Observe as the detached witness of action. God is the do-er, God is the observer, and you are THAT.

ATMA VIDYA ASHRAM

"WE need to feed the poor children in India," stated Swamini Lalitananda shortly after arriving in our home.

"How can we do that? I responded.

"We should start an *ashram* and feed them."

So began my new assignment of helping Swamini Lalitananda with her mission of feeding the poor children in India. The *Atma Vidya* (knowledge of our divinity) *Ashram* was given its name by Swami Dayananda at the *Arsha Vidya Gurukulum* after we had proposed our plan to him. We had to fund this project and get the funds to India in a way that assured that we were indeed, feeding the poor children of India. We incorporated in the year 2000 and began teaching yoga, philosophy and Hinduism to whomever showed interest. After a challenging first year, Swamiji joined forces with another Swami of the Sivananda lineage to operate the orphanages in India. Swami Omananda became the India counterpart and Swamini Lalitananda worked the United States I held down the "corporate ashram" in our home. We developed a schedule of travel and teaching as well as direct mail campaign that raised thousands of dollars. The India Development and Relief Fund matched donations we got, so rupees started flowing to feed the poor children of India. Chuck and I traveled to Bangalore India to meet Swami Omananda and see first hand how things were going.

"It's like swimming through a sea of little boys," said my dear husband. "They're everywhere."

Needless to say, we fell in love with our boys. They called us "Divya Aunty" and "Chuck Uncle" and followed us everywhere. They loved our digital camera and especially loved Chuck Uncle's hat. One of the most endearing things was their desire to serve us food.

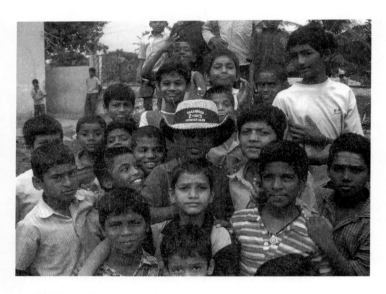

"Just orange juice," said a modest Chuck Uncle. After what seemed like an hour, we realized that to provide us with "just orange juice" Swami Omananda had to dig up rupees for the boys to run into the village with their bare feet, to buy oranges. Met at the entrance by other boys, the oranges got peeled and squeezed by many loving and probably dirty little hands.

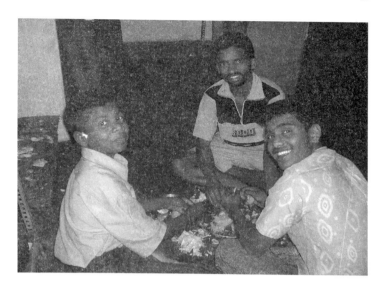

We had been "sponsoring" a young boy of the ashram for a year by this time. Swami Omananda agreed that we could take him and another boy with us to Sai Baba's Ashram and that Omananda himself would love to come too. Off we went with our hired car and driver to Puttaparthi singing bhajans and very happy.

"Turn here," shouted Swami Omananda to our driver.

"NO," responded Chuck. "I want to be in Puttaparthi to receive Baba's darshan. We can't detour!'

"Just a short stop," said a smiling Omananda and we soon found ourselves in a little dusty village. Word spread like wild fire down the ally ways of the village.

"OMANANDA IS HERE,
OMANANDA IS HERE."

We were escorted into a stucco hut and offered tea by a lovely young woman whose family had known Omananda for years. Our visit was filled with love and tenderness. With no expectations for an outcome, we surrendered to the moment.

Hours later, we found ourselves in Puttaparthi at Sai Baba's ashram in time for the darshan of Sathya Sai Baba, but Omananda received a phone call and had to leave for Bangalore.

"But why? We both asked? We were told, "the rice did not arrive."

Bewildered, we asked, "What do you mean?" It seems that the man who promised to donate rice to the orphanage did not come. There was no food for the boys. The ashram houses over 125 boys and a handful of destitute women. No rice meant that there wouldn't be dinner. We called for the driver and Swami Omananda sped away beginning a three-hour drive back to Bangalore. You see? He had no expectation of reward or recognition. He gave up his stay in Sai Baba's presence and did his duty. He did it for love and only love. This is how we make our future by popping the seeds of *karma*! We make our future by popping the seeds of *karma* with love.

KARMA

KARMA is a word that we hear about more and more in the west. It pretty much means, "As you sow, so shall you reap." If you plant poor seeds, then you grow bad crops. I remember hearing once that karma was like seeds stored in a large silo. The seeds from many seasons get stored in that silo. The seeds that are pulled out of the bottom may be several seasons old. The farmer might not remember if that was a good growing year or not, but the seeds got harvested and placed in the silo. "What goes around, comes around," is another way of looking at karma. Good begets good, and bad begets bad.

I have no control over the seeds that are already stored in my psyche. I came into this world with certain genes, skills, abilities, and weaknesses. These are all karmic seeds that I have no control over in this birth and neither do you. Did you choose the country of your birth, or the family that you were born into? Did you choose your skin color, looks or physical impairment? Why can't I be smarter, prettier, loved more, stronger, and more athletically inclined? We were born this way and there isn't anything that we can do about that.

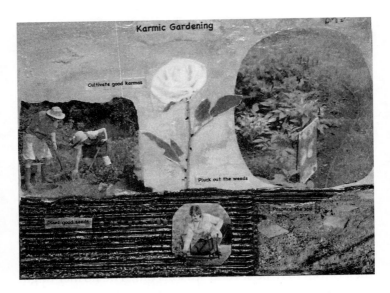

Chuck and I had both been brought up in the Catholic faith. We had belonged to the same church. So attending an Easter vigil at our local Catholic church was comfortable for me. Chuck warned me that as divorced people, we no longer belonged there, but this was before we had been led to a more Eastern philosophy, so off I went. Every day for a week I participated fully in the prayers and healing masses. On the fourth session, I was praying and holding the intent that these healing prayers would help me to be a good mother to our five children. Blending a family is a challenge and meeting the needs of these children of divorce was tricky parenting.

After mass, I left the church by the side door and headed to my car to drive home. As I inserted the key in the ignition, the front windshield of the car lit up. Brilliant white light radiated into the car and I heard the words "Chuck's children are your children!" My head dropped to the wheel and I started to cry. In that moment, I was fully aware that this was karma. I had lost three babies during my married years before meeting Chuck. Having grown up with five siblings, I had hoped for a larger family. *Karmically*, the souls of the three babies that I could not provide a full term body for were already embodied. These three perfect souls were the children that Chuck brought to our marriage. I didn't choose these children: they came with the marriage. There was a bigger picture, a movie drama being played out and I was playing the role of mother.

That happened 35 years ago. Since then, Chuck's first wife has passed away. I play the role of loving, supportive parent to all of our five children and our nine beautiful grandchildren. Seeds planted lifetimes ago have come to fruition.

What I do in this life is what creates the *karmas* of tomorrow. It is in my best interest to plant good seeds in this lifetime. This *karmic* gardening is important for practicing the 8 limbs of yoga. We need to be aware of the seeds that we are planting and cultivating. We need to be mindful of the weeds in our *karmic* garden and pull them out while they are still little and weak. If we allow these little weeds to take hold, they grow into *kleshas* (negative thought waves) that give rise to afflictions and miseries.

None of us wants to suffer in this lifetime. But the Buddha tells us that life is suffering. How can we manage these thought waves so that we don't suffer? *Karmic* gardening is the yogic technique for managing these thoughts that plague the mind. Pull out the weeds. Can you even recognize the weeds from the good *karmic* plants? Plant good seeds. Seeds of love, compassion, self-confidence, serenity, friendliness,and cheerfulness. Recognize these as they grow in your personality. Recognize the weeds as they sprout and pull them up and out! One weed that may try to take hold, is anger. Being angry can take years off your life and create more *karma*, if you act on it. Don't let it take root. We can catch ourself and transform any harmful emotion. Greed is another example of a weed that we should transform. Plant seeds of generosity. The more you give, the more you get. Do you want love? You can never grow love if you plant seeds of hate. Plant compassion. If little weeds of judgement or intolerance sprout, weed the garden and become aware of how your thoughts can create happiness or negativity in your life.

REINCARNATION

ABOUT thirty years ago, Chuck and I decided to ask Bob, a friend who had been trained in hypnosis, to regress me. If Chuck and I were really soul mates, then we figured we must have had other lives together. Prior to the session, Chuck and I listed the names of family members and some questions that we wanted answered during the regression. I sat comfortably on my couch and Bob started counting me backward, as if I were riding backward on a train and watching the years slip by. He said if there was any time I wanted to stop, just raise my hand. At one point, he stopped and asked me if I had any recall, emotions or feelings. I responded that it was dark and I had the sensation of bugs, big black bugs.

On we went back in time until I raised my hand again and Bob started asking me questions. I can tell you what I remember seeing at that time. I realized that I was seeing myself as a male Native American. I wore skins on my lower body and feet. I "saw" a bear in the river catching fish with his claws. I hid my canoe under some brush. I was fearful about the white men who lived in a house made of wood. I refused to look in the windows when Bob encouraged me to do so. I was frightened of them. Chuck encouraged Bob to ask me about the people in that life. So names of family in this life were mentioned and I shook my head "no" to all of my children and my husband and even my parents in this life. None were with me in the Native American life, until he mentioned my sister Susan.

Sue, was my best friend, another male Indian. My sister Jeri was there too, as my squaw. I answered "yes' that I had children and named two of them but could not name the baby in my arms. According to Chuck's recollection, I spoke in an animated fashion using signs. When my brother Drew's name was mentioned, I got extremely agitated recalling a battle scene where my brother was killed. When asked what that life's lesson was for me, I answered, "The chief is not always right."

I was brought out of the hypnosis session with the suggestion that when Bob said a certain word, I would get up, wash my hands and offer him a drink. And sure enough, I found myself following those directions.

Chuck went immediately to the telephone and called my mother. He asked her "Mom, when you were in Texas, pregnant with Patty, were there any bugs there?" My mother's answer was "Oh my God. Bugs, big black bugs, everywhere!" Those bugs were swarms of locust-like insects. She'd never mentioned this to me. It seemed that I had recall from between lives, in utero.

The next day, both Bob and Chuck did some research on Native American tribes to verify my remembrances. They documented the area of the United States that I said I lived, the style of dwelling that I said we lived in, and the fact that we did not have horses or hunt buffalo. I started thinking back to my sisters and their younger years. My sister Susan changed the spelling of her name to Sioux and wore her hair in braids with a leather thong around her forehead; my sister Jeri was into making Indian crafts. In this current lifetime, I have always challenged authority. Maybe that's because "the chief is not always right."

KLESHAS

THE *kleshas* are really just bad thoughts. There are five main *kleshas* that seem to really bog us down when it comes to keeping our *karmic* garden free from weeds. The first one is **ignorance**. This doesn't mean limited knowledge of worldly things; it means ignorance of our connection to God. We think that we are separate, when in reality, we are ONE. The second one is **egoism**. By egoism I mean that the more we think that our minds and bodies are who we really are. We get pretty puffed up or greatly let down depending on how we perceive our bodies. The spiritual truth is that we are not physical beings occasionally getting a glimpse of spirit; we are spiritual beings having a physical existence. We are not the body or the brain. We are pure spirit, experiencing life in this body with this brain. The third *klesha* is **attachment**. If our minds become too attached to anything, then we will suffer when that thing disappears. Think about losing something that you are extremely attached to: children, home, car, pet, partner. If they are gone tomorrow, we suffer great loss. We strive to cultivate unconditional love for all. By being accepting of the way things are, we no longer try to control the way we want things to be. To love with no conditions is challanging. The closer we are to a person, the more expectations we have of that person. Unconditional love is accepting with no condition and no expectations. The fourth *klesha* is **hatred**. Nothing makes more space between God and us than hatred. We examine our reaction toward things and strive to be neutral, if not loving. A strong emotion such as hatred builds a wall between us and whatever it is we hate. If our goal is to attain unity, union with our god-source, there is no room for hatred. All things, no matter how we perceive them in form, are divine in essence. The fifth *klesha* **is fear of death**. Most people have a fear of the unknown. That deep, dark void is the ultimate unknown.

If we can remove the *kleshas* of ignorance, egoism, attachment and hatred from our mind, what is there to fear? Death becomes simply the changing of one's clothes. We slip out of our current body and move onward as a body of light. If we have been successful in destroying these *kleshas* or negative thought waves, we have popped the seeds of *karma*. If we have popped the seeds of *karma*, they can no longer bear fruit. Think good thoughts. Create loving thought waves and experience a life filled with self-confidence and security. Be friendly and cheerful to others and they will reflect these qualities right back to you.

Our thoughts are very powerful. I have found that we can think of what we want in life and make that thought come true. It takes follow-through: making a plan, setting goals and carrying out the activities that will help us reach our goal. Thoughts can be our downfall as well. When we let our mind control us with negative thoughts, we manifest that negativity in our lives. "Are we that powerful?" you may ask. I believe that we all are. Those thought waves are called *vrittis* in Sanskrit. They are always coming and going, flitting through the mind like butterflies. It's very difficult to stop them but we can decide which ones our mind will engage and which ones to let pass right through.

Years ago, I became friendly with Addie, a wise older woman in her nineties who lived in Florida. Addie had a funny philosophical directive for negative thought waves. She'd say, "Quit your stinkin thinkin." How profound this simple statement really is. When we are fearful, thoughts of what may happen flood our mind. It scares us until we are paralyzed. The antidote to this is to quit our "stinkin thinkin" as Addie would say. These things are not really happening to us. They are only happening in our mind. If we can dismiss these negative thought forms and engage in positive action, we can create a beautiful, positive world for ourselves. We DO create our own reality, every minute of every day. Let the beautiful butterflies light in your mind and create a beautiful day.

Bad things do happen. How can we not react? How can we not be so totally wrapped up in the sad drama that we become depressed. Try to remember that life is like a movie drama. We are the cast. Imagine that you were cast as the mother in this particular movie. Good actors can cry on cue. They may have to shoot a scene over and over again, but they don't get depressed or suicidal over it. They detach from the drama when their workday is over. Somebody else has written the script, so the actor learns the lines and plays that character to the best of his/her ability. Some acting is so fine, that we find ourselves feeling the emotion, crying or fearfully covering our eyes just watching the drama. But when the movie is over, we detach from those emotions and go on with our life.

Knowing how to play the role in which we are cast in this lifetime can be a challenge. We don't have written scripts and can't talk to the director, or can we? Prayer and meditation can help. When one of our children had become addicted to alcohol, I was devastated. Fear and attachment paralyzed me. Finally, I resorted to morning meditations on this family drama. Every morning, before dawn, I would sit in meditation out on our deck before the family awakened. I asked for guidance as I would if I were talking to the director of the movie. I really didn't know what to do with this fourteen-year old child whose genetic pre-disposition had contributed to this situation. Then one morning, I heard the words "Call your insurance company." I didn't know that God, the cosmic director knew anything about insurance companies, but I followed this sage advice. One call led to another and then an appointment, then in-patient treatment. This child is now an adult, has never had another drink, and has helped countless people with addiction issues. Is this karma playing out? I like to think that he is popping the seeds of karma so he does not have to come back and do this again.

There is a story in the "recovery" world about walking down a road and falling into a huge pothole. We get all banged up and it may take some time to pull ourselves out of the hole. The next time we walk down that road, we see the hole and are convinced we won't slip again, but sure enough, we do. The next time, we give ourselves a wide birth by walking on the other side of the street, but it happens again and again. How can we avoid this pothole? By taking another road! Robert Frost says "and I took the road less traveled by and that has made all the difference." Sometimes, in order to change, something must change, or nothing changes. That 'something' needs to be us. Stop doing the same old things expecting life to change. Pull out the karmic weeds, those attributes in our personality that are creating misery in your life. Our son did just that. He broke the cycle by taking another road. He climbed the twelve steps by working the steps one by one. He moved from a dark, *tamasic* state to an active, *rajasic* life filled with helping others. Twenty-five years later, he still sponsors men in recovery from substance abuse and helps them reach the twelfth step in their program. Twelve-step programs are very spiritual and if followed diligently, can lead to God Realization.

My friend Mac used to use our house overlooking the river, to do step work with the men he sponsored. He felt that to get and stay sober and follow a twelve-step program was a surefire way to burn the *karmic* seeds of addiction and reach God Realization. After years of living in a dumpster and shooting heroin, Mac got straight and found his way to an *ashram*, the home of a spiritual monk. It was by total surrender to his guru and God that he was able to continue to follow the twelve-step path and lead other addicts to it. Mac was not doing this for a reward of any kind. As a matter of fact, many of the people he sponsored, fell back into addiction and just disappeared.

"No attachment to the outcome," he'd bellow.

"Just do what ya gotta do, one day at a time."

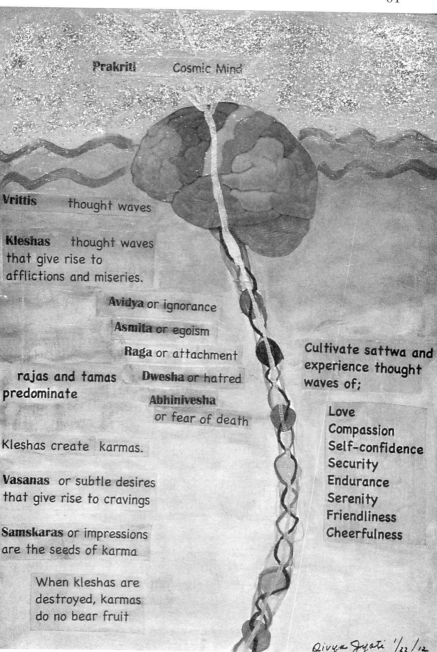

Prakriti   Cosmic Mind

Vrittis   thought waves

Kleshas   thought waves
that give rise to
afflictions and miseries.

Avidya or ignorance

Asmita or egoism

Raga or attachment

rajas and tamas   **Dwesha** or hatred
predominate

Abhinivesha
or fear of death

Cultivate sattwa and
experience thought
waves of;

Love
Compassion
Self-confidence
Security
Endurance
Serenity
Friendliness
Cheerfulness

Kleshas create karmas.

Vasanas or subtle desires
that give rise to cravings

Samskaras or impressions
are the seeds of karma

When kleshas are
destroyed, karmas
do no bear fruit

Divya Jyoti ¹/₂₂/₁₂

"But how do you do it Mac," I'd ask and he'd answer, "Ya fake it till ya make it."

Controlling our thoughts is how we fake it. Our thoughts may keep returning to those things that we have become addicted to, be it drink, drugs, pills, sex or food. Yet, we must redirect our thoughts from those addictions to positive thoughts.

Mac would try to get the people that he was sponsoring to change their thoughts from their craving to something else. He'd encourage them to "Call a friend! Call me!" He knew that if they changed their thoughts, they could change their lives.

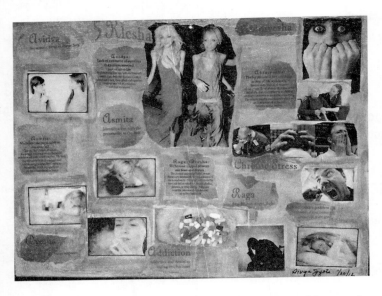

"Surrender to a higher power." Mac would preach. Know that while you are alone and powerless, with the help of that higher power, you can resist the pull of

addictive thoughts and desires. Mac was under no delu-
sions. He'd tell you that he was an addict. Even though
it had been decades since he was active as an addict. But
this man moved through the stages of *tamas* (sloth-drug
use) to *rajas* (action-changing his thoughts) to *sattwa*
(peace). The sweetness and light that emerged from Mac
was pure love, compassion, and serenity. He oozed self-
confidence without being cocky. Mac died as a result of
the years of abuse. Although hepatitis took him, when he
passed, he was clutching his prayer beads and repeating
his *mantra* and concentrating on the God within.

It's a good time now to re-examine *kleshas* or negative thoughts and what we do with them. *Kleshas* are
thought waves of ego, attachment, hatred and fear, and
these thoughts are what create the weeds of *karma* in our
garden of life. Can you recognize these in your garden? It
takes awareness to see these thought waves and change
them. When *kleshas* are destroyed, negative *karmas* bear
no fruit. This is how we pull out the weeds and cut down
the trees of worldly passions.

Kleshas or dark thoughts that give way to misery and
afflictions grow out of a *tamasic* lifestyle. I remember
how terrible I felt in my younger days after a night of
partying. My head hurt, my stomach hurt, and I didn't
want to go anywhere. I just wanted to sleep. And some
days, I did just that. We cannot aspire to a yogic lifestyle
by being *tamasic*. I was very lucky that my *tamasic* lifestyle at that time did not result in major *kleshas*. With
addictions in my family, I came into this world with
those *karmic* seeds. It would be very easy to get stuck in

those *vasana* (subtle desires) that give way to cravings. Giving in to those cravings creates *samskaras*. I think of *samskaras* as ruts. I picture a stagecoach with those big wooden wheels bumbling down a dirt road. The wheels make ruts and the wagon wants to stay traveling in those ruts. In order to get out of the rut, we need to make a lot of effort. Even if we manage to steer ourselves out of the rut, if we are not mindful, we slip right back into it. So we need to move from a life of *tamas* to a life of *rajas* (activity or passion). Get up and get going.

Finding happiness in things outside of you is to chase the illusory butterfly of life. The more we desire something, the more we need to fulfill our desires. This mentality of "I need more" can kill us. We may feel that if this feels good, more will make me feel even better. This could be desire for self-gratification or just greed in general. There is a difference between feeling good and contentment. More money, bigger houses or fancy cars may make us feel good and feed our egos but these things don't bring contentment. Often times they bring more darkness and fear. We worry and stress out about losing the big house or cry over totaling the luxury car. We may fear life itself as a scary place, and that separation from who we really are, creates an irrational fear of death as well. Remember, *kleshas* are thought waves that lead to misery and affliction. Dr. Wayne Dyer talks about changing our thoughts in his famous book *Change Your Thoughts: Change Your Life*. Sounds easy, doesn't it? But when you are in a rut, it's hard to pull yourself out of it. Knowing the difference between wants, desires and needs is an important realization.

GUNAS – PERSONALITY CHARACTERISTICS

Do something…anything…just keep your mind out of the rut. Stay focused on something positive. I did service to others. My career involved helping others. I worked for a community action agency and it felt good to go to work and make a difference. I learned that the foods I ate helped me get out of the darkness and into an active lifestyle. By eliminating alcohol and red meat, I felt less tamasic, lethargic, dark, and lazy. By eating Indian foods with those tasty spices, I got charged up and wanted to do things. I became passionate about making a difference. I remember once organizing a Five Minutes of Silence demonstration in front of the soup kitchen in downtown Middletown against drug and alcohol abuse. Hundreds of people from all walks of life showed up. We made the front page of the city newspaper. I stood holding hands with my teenage son, my lawyer husband, homeless people and Head Start preschoolers in silence, for five long minutes. Words were not needed. We all knew what we were fighting, and we knew that addiction is a rut that is easy to fall back into. Don't walk down that path folks, take another route. The route I chose was to live a yogic life, which led me to practicing a more satwic lifestyle. Satwa is harmony and purity.

One day soon after the *Five Minutes of Silence* demonstration, a grizzly old ex heroin addict came into my office to talk me into starting a "Food Share" program. You guessed it! It was Mac, about whom I spoke a few pages back. He had seen this type of thing in other states, and knew of one in Willimantic. He was persuasive and I found myself renting a box truck and driving to Willimantic on a cold autumn morning to pick up fresh fruits and vegetables to distribute to the poor. Mac knew it wasn't enough to live free from alcohol and drugs. We all need to move from tamas through *rajas* to *satwa*. Fresh fruits and vegetables are pure, healthy, living, *satwic* foods. What better service could there be than to help poor families feed themselves fresh, affordable produce? This program became so popular that we had hundreds of people lining up monthly for a box of fresh food in dozens of church parking lots across the state. Cultivate *satwa* and experience thought waves of love, compassion, self-confidence, security, endurance, serenity, friendliness and cheerfulness. The "share team" grew and was soon running on it's own. People were cooperating, smiling and self–confident. In the course of evolution, the gross oil of *tamas* must be converted into the active *rajas,* ascending the wick and then, sublimated into the luminous flame of *satwa*.

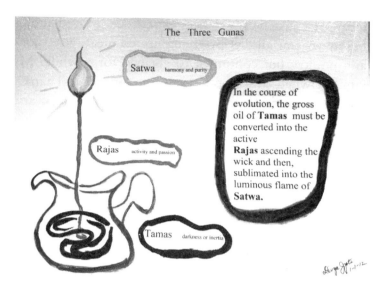

The Three Gunas

Satwa harmony and purity

Rajas activity and passion

In the course of evolution, the gross oil of **Tamas** must be converted into the active **Rajas** ascending the wick and then, sublimated into the luminous flame of **Satwa.**

Tamas darkness or inertia

Foods contribute to the *gunas* (the characteristics) that we present in our personalities. Eating meat, smoking, drinking alcohol, and taking drugs make our bodies dark, lethargic and *tamasic*. Eating spicy foods, sugar, caffeine and the like, tend to speed up our metabolism and give us *rajasic* passion. This passion can be a zest for life and get you going. Substituting *rajasic* foods like a nice spicy curry rather than foods like a 2-day-old pizza, will get you moving in a hurry. But better still, is to move from stimulating foods to *satwic* foods. Fresh fruits, vegetables, dairy products, nuts, and whole grains make our personalities more balanced. The more pure the food we consume, the more *sattwic* or pure our nature becomes. I have been a vegetarian for over 30 years now. Having been brought up by a large, loving Italian family, giving up meatballs and sausage was quite an effort. My mother-in-law especially had trouble with us not eating meat. She just didn't understand it. We moved into a purely vegetarian diet by giving up red meat, veal, pork and poultry but continued to eat fish for a while. My family owned a seafood restaurant and one Thanksgiving, swordfish steaks were prepared for Chuck and me, because we didn't eat turkey. I'll never forget that Thanksgiving. I could not stand the smell of that fish. I handed the whole plate of nicely grilled swordfish to Chuck. That's when I knew that I had turned the bend in my eating patterns. My *guru* told us that when an animal is slaughtered, all of the fear in the animal is released into the flesh. If we eat that flesh, we ingest that energy. As a practitioner of *ahimsa* (non-violence) I have no desire whatsoever, to consume any form of flesh ever again.

MEDITATION

methods to control the mind
and direct Divine Energy

A M I living my yoga yet? Am I practicing off the mat, so to speak? When we purifiy our thoughts, words and deeds, lots of other stuff can come up. We are complex systems after all. A study of the chakras (Energy points along the spine) helped me to understand what was happening in meditation. I was meditating regularly with a wonderful teacher at the Hindu Temple in Middletown for at least an hour per session. Often I would experience uncontrollable shaking and moving while in meditation. I started to study the seven chakras (energy vortexes)and kundalini shakti (movement of energy in the body). My teacher helped me learn how to control this energy and allow it to ascend to the crown chakra. In my years of practice, I've moved slowly in being able to purify the nadis (energy channels) so that my physical body and mind could hold this energy. Concentration, contemplation and meditation, and going within, help me to quiet my mind.

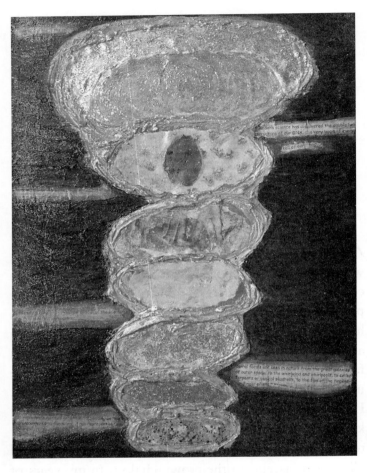

Many times in meditation, I would experience spiral energy. Sometimes I would be IN that spiral. It felt kind of like Alice from Alice in Wonderland falling down the rabbit hole. I'd see different colors too. Quite the psychedelic trips those early meditations. Sometimes, I would be spiraling upward and could sense the energy becoming more subtle. It was many years later, while teaching about the *chakras,* that I made the connection between my "spiral meditations," and the *kundalini* energy rising through the *chakras.*

Pranayam

Pranayama is essential for meditation and going within as is living a pure lifestyle of practicing the *yamas* and the *niyamas.* I define *prana* as Divine Life Force, the energy that keeps us alive. When we breathe, *prana* rides on the breath. *Prana* circulates through the body and keeps our organs functioning. Imagine a person who had been involved in a terrible accident. Imagine their heart stopped beating and they were shocked back only to lose consciousness and be placed on life support. If *prana* has left the body, all the machines available cannot bring life back, even if the heart is pumping, lungs expanding and contracting etc. Nobody is home. We refer to this as brain dead. The energy body *(pranamaya kosha)* has vacated the body. Building this *prana* in our bodies helps us to heal and keeps us healthy. There are many different *pranayamas* that yogis practice. The easiest and most profound in my opinion, is alternate nostril breathing. My guru taught me that this technique is the safest way possible by inhaling through the left nostril and exhaling through the right nostril. This soothing breath cools the body and is easy on the nervous system. I moved from this to alternating nostrils thus activating the *ida* and the *pingala nadis,* which are the pathways that energy travels on either side of the spinal column in the energetic body. I also practice cleansing breaths such as forceful exhalations through alternate nostrils. Nice full 3 part yogic breaths help us to expand lung capacity and build tolerance for *pranayam*. Building up slowly allows us to activate the *kundalini* energy at the base of the spine in the energetic body. If we don't have a steady gradual practice of *pranayam*, our physical bodies will have difficulty holding this energy.

Kundalini

Kundalini is a Sanskrit word that translates to coiled serpent. The energy that runs through our body is sometimes referred to as *kundalini* energy because some seers have likened it to a snake moving upward. When this energy starts to move up the *shushumna*, (the major energy pathway in the center of the spinal column,) it snakes its way through the energy centers referred to as *chakras*, or energy vortexes. If the body is not purified and strong enough to hold this energy, strange things may occur. I have heard it said that when we die, we want our *pranic* body to exit through the crown of our head, not through a lower *chakra*. So, what better way to prepare to leave our body, then to leave the body through a *kundalini* experience. This energy moves from the root *chakra* in the base of the spine, traverses the *chakras* and exits at the crown of the head. In a sexual experience, this energy is stimulated and we have a very pleasant experience. Just imagine how pleasant this experience would be if we could hold the energy until it exits the crown *chakra*.

One visit to India tested my physical ability to hold this energy. My friend Linda and I were doing a program at the nearby *ayurvedic* clinic and returning to the *ashram* every afternoon. These *ayurvedic* sessions included hot oil massages, fasting, herbal enemas and special *ayurvedic* herbal teas and were extremely purifying. That treatment, coupled with the purity of living in an *ashram* prepared me for a unique experience. While meditating one afternoon at Sai Baba's ashram, my body started shaking. The shaking was especially prevalent in my neck and head. I had no control over these jerky movements. Then I experienced my body levitating off the bed that I was sitting on. I tried to call to my friend Linda, but nothing but mumbled, garbled grunts came out of my mouth. Linda was in the bathroom and unable to respond to my call. Finally, several minutes later, she came into my room and sat behind me. She placed her hands on my shoulders and gently brought me back into my body.

She grounded me through her hands on my shoulders and regulated her breathing with mine to bring me back into my body consciousness.

This energy can get knotted in various organs and parts of the body causing distress. It is best to practice these techniques with the guidance of an experienced teacher.

I levitated another time on the deck of my home. I had recently returned from a trip to Sai Baba's ashram in India (I've been there 10 times) and was meditating on my cushion outside on my deck. As I opened my eyes to gaze out to the river, I noticed that one of the trees in my line of vision was sinking. I reached down to my meditation cushion and it was right under me but both the cushion and I were elevated. The tree wasn't sinking, I was lifting!

I have been involved in organizing silent, meditation

and yoga retreats since the early 1990's. These retreats, away from my work and family routine allow me to really experience divinity not only within me as in deep meditation, but also around me. Of course I lead *yoga asana* classes at these retreats but I also get to take silent walks in nature that open me up to experiencing God in everything, the trees foliage, the flowers, the little bunnies and squirrels, the sky and the placid lake. Everything seemed alive in God. I'd like to share some of my experiences during these retreats from my journals.

Oct. 15, 1994
"I'm here at St. Mary's Villa for a peaceful three days of silence. It's very beautiful here with the foliage all orange and gold and red. We took a brisk walk this morning with the Buddhist gong. Every minute or so, our leader would hit the gong. We would then stop, focus on the moment, then continue. It was quite a dramatic experience for me. Once, when we stopped, I felt a rush of energy go through me and out the top of my head. I was so overcome, tears came to my eyes. As I walked on again, the orange trees seemed brighter. Everything appeared to have more depth and vividness to it. Experiencing God within while maintaining silence is quite profound. I'm in a constant state of meditation- always."

Oct.16, 1994
This meditation is dizzying! I'm on another plane altogether. I lost it twice during mantra chanting.

God only knows where I was. When I came back everyone else was gone. I experienced the descent of the 'holy spirit' in meditation. A white bird came down, head first over and through my head. I saw a soft white light, cover my head and shoulders. The bird became more like a ghost as it passed down through my body. The almost translucent white enveloped me and brought total peace.

Oct.17, 1994

I experienced a total single- pointed ness in meditation this morning. A rainbow colored column appeared- very thin and off centered. It adjusted itself in my forehead area until it was centered. Then from the back of my head, I felt a buzz-ing feeling. The buzz came through my head and focused on the rainbow column. I was able to hold onto this sensation for quite a while.

June 11,1996

Prindle Pond, MA

Nadine lead a guided meditation and had us working with "love energy." I pictured a soft pink pulsating energy in the room outside and in front of me. Then I saw a large white lotus flower in the middle of the room. The lotus began pulsat-ing. The outer petals began moving slowly up and down. Nadine was saying something about send-ing love energy around the world, when from the middle of the flower a fountain of white sparks started to shoot up into the universe. I had the

experience of this energy being so strong that it
was not limited to the earth. I felt a large white
energy come toward me from the lotus and just
melt across and into my body. I felt very warm
and peaceful. My breathing was shallow...almost
non-existent...such peace, love and bliss. Then,
I felt like I was going to sneeze. My conscious
thought was NO, not now! Suddenly, the sensation of sneezing went up through my head and
felt like it had blown the top half of my head right
off. The energy changed in my body dramatically.
My heart began pounding like a jack- hammer. I
could feel the blood, flowing through my veins.
The energy was so intense I didn't think my body
could withstand it. SOMETHING was witnessing
this occurring in my body but it wasn't really me.
"I" was blown out through the top of my head
into a world of color the likes of which I could
never imagine. Vivid oranges, gold and purple
colors surrounded me and I existed as a heavy,
liquid, flowing syrupy golden substance, like lava.
It took quite a while for me to come back totally.
I was aware of Nadine calling my name but I
couldn't move. "I" in the form of Patty wanted to
respond but the "I" that was the golden lava was
pretty content. When I finally got grounded, I was
extremely warm and spacey.

July 30,1996
I was in a beautiful villa helping run an orphanage
with the nuns. Our nun's habits were saris. I was

told to follow sister Maria and do whatever she did. Sai Baba came and we all followed him. We started rolling down a grassy slope. I was rolling in my sari, fabric flying, when suddenly I was face to face with Sai Baba. I looked happily into his eyes. His face was as bright as the sun, but there was a white gossamer veil between his face and mine.

"Oh," I cried..."I wish that this were real."

"Oh, but it is" he said.

"No really, Baba, I wish that I could stay here with you forever".

He looked pensively to one side then said.

"You help, and some day you will be with me forever."

It was almost five years later that I met and began to help Swamini Lalitananda who wears the orange sari of a renuciate. I continue to help her support orphanages to feed and educate destitute children in India.

The Genie

There is an interesting story that I tell in my *yoga* classes about a poor young man in India trying to eke a living out of the barren soil. While digging in the field, he unearthed a lamp. Rubbing the lamp with his shirt, a genie appeared to him and granted him three wishes. The young man was amazed at his good fortune and immediately asked that his field be fertile and produce a rich crop. Bam! His wish was granted.

"Give me something to do, or I will destroy you," said

the genie. The young man asked for a decent home for his family and BAM! His wish was granted.

"Give me something to do, or I will destroy you," said the genie. The young man thought hard this time. He had all that he needed. But he was worried that this genie might destroy him, so for his third wish, he asked the genie to create a tall pole and climb up to the top and slide down to the bottom and keep doing this.

"I will do as you say," said the genie. He continued to climb up and down the pole and the young man lived happily ever after.

The symbolism in this story is not easy to understand. The genie represents our mind. It can create a wonderful world for us, but an idle mind can cause problems. If we do not keep it occupied, it can destroy us. Remember the *kleshas*? They are the negative thought waves that give way to afflictions and miseries. The pole represents the *shushumna* or the energy pathway that runs up the spinal cord. Moving up and down the pole is the *prana* that rides on the breath. When we focus our mind in meditation, we regulate our breath and *pranic* energy moves smoothly upward creating a blissful state of meditation.

The Lotus

Yogis often use the lotus flower as a symbol of meditation. I love this image and whenever I see a peaceful pond with a lotus (lily pad), I try to take a photo of it or sketch it to remind me that although we have our roots in the world, we can aspire to the heights of detachment in meditation. The lotus flower sinks its roots into the muddy bottom of the pond. Slowly it grows upward, through the mucky water. This stem is like the *shushumna.*(energy channel in the middle of the spinal column) The stem strives to reach the surface of the water where it blossoms beautifully in the sunlight. The lotus flower sits on the lily pad and does not even touch the mucky waters of this world. As we strive to perfect our meditation, we too can rise up through the energy centers that govern our bodily functions in this world, to the crown chakra, and realize the bliss of our true nature.

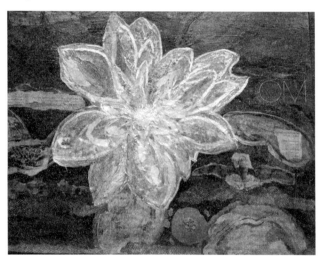

Japa and Mantra

An interesting technique for keeping the mind peaceful and connected to the divine, is called *japa*. This is the repetition of a *mantra* or a name of God like Jesus, Buddha, Sai etc, 108 times. Sitting with a straight spine, moving my fingers over my *japa mala* beads, I would go into a blissful state by just repeating the *mantra* and riding the waves of vibration. *Japa* is like "priming the pump" for me and I find if I do it, I sink into a very deep meditative state. The deep breathing and prayerful intent starts to move that divine *prana* until the mind is focused only on the *mantra*. All thought waves that bring us outward, are calmed. The *mantra* begins to repeat in my mind automatically. I sometimes go to sleep doing *japa* and wake up repeating the *mantra*. I've programmed in the divine name and deleted the files that are not needed in my brain to surrender to the blissful divine vibe.

As a Catholic, I used to say the rosary. In times of distress, like when my grandson had cancer, my daughter and I would say the rosary together. It's really the same idea.

OM: The Divine in the form of sound

Chanting the sound of *Om* (pronounced A-U-M) is a very powerful practice. I find it most effective as a daily morning mantra done in a seated posture with a straight aligned spine. Begin by breathing deeply. My guru taught us that the sound of Ahh starts deep in the navel region and comes up to the throat. He said to picture an airplane on the runway, ready to take off. As the sound comes up into the throat, let the mouth open to form an O shape. Now the sound is like a plane right overhead. Bring the lips together to create a vibration as the sound Mmm leaves from your sealed lips. This is like the plane leaving our sight. Feel the Mmm sound in the center of your forehead. Take another deep breath and repeat this pattern. The sacred sound of *Om* can be chanted any number of times but the most powerful number of times is nine, eighteen, 108, or any multiple of 9 (Nine is the numeric symbol of infinite divinity). An easy way to count the repetitions is to use a *japa mala* or rosary. *Om* is the sound of the universe. It's the hum or vibration of creation. "From the sound of silence, came the voice of God. *Om, Om, Om, Hari Om.* "

The chanting of *Omkar* is one of my favorite spiritual practices in the *ashram* or at a retreat. A large group of people gathers in silence just before dawn to sit in silent meditation. The harmonium starts its drone. A collective breath is drawn in and out comes the breath of God in the sound of *Om.* This continues for 108 times. The room is electrified with divine energy. You can feel the vibration in your body and on your lips and in the Third Eye in the middle of your forehead. Ending with *"shanti, shanti, shantihi"* (peace, peace, peace,) the room falls silent and we sink into a deep meditation.

Chakras – Energy Centers in the Body

There have been tons of books written about the *chakras*. If you want to make a study of them, I recommend the books and tapes of Anodea Judith available at Sounds True publishing. I see the *chakras* as spinning energy vortexes. The practice of yoga helps to open these energy centers and align us with our true nature. Most yoga teachers can help you find postures that can help remove blockages and open the *chakras*. I find that a class that combines pranic breathing, stretching, twisting, and focusing inward can usually bring a yoga student into an awareness of where energy is stuck in his/her body. I often guide students inward to experience the body and the emotions that may arise during certain postures. I spend a fair bit of time on the lower *chakras* because many students of yoga are very much "in" their bodies but not necessarily aware of their bodies other than outward appearances.

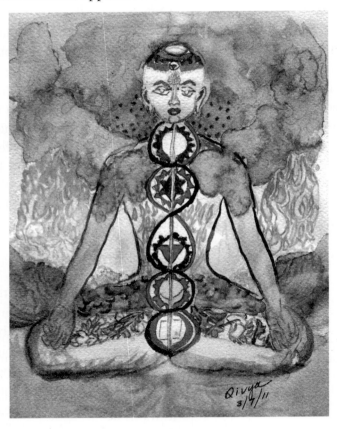

A focus on the root *chakra* and postures for the legs, help us come to terms with issues of belonging both to this planet and to our community. We do grounding postures and sink imaginary roots into mother earth. Second *chakra* issues often relate to women's issues. Emotional wounds can be experienced and released. Third *chakra* issues can relate to will power. Developing strength and experiencing one's power is related to this fire in the belly. The fourth *chakra* energy is subtler. As we move spiritual awareness into the heart *chakra*, we can experience a sense of love and compassion. I'd like to share one little story about my experience opening the heart *chakra*.

Many years ago I attended a program at the *Kripalu* Center in Lenox MA. Back in those days, *Kripalu* was an *ashram*. Yogi Amrit DeSai was the head of the *ashram* and was teaching this course. We did a variety of *asana* and many of them were held for long periods of time. I don't remember which ones were used but I will never forget the result. By the end of this class with Gurudev, my heart *chakra* was wide open. How do I know that my heart *chakra* was opened? First of all, I felt unconditional love in that moment. My chest felt expansive and full. Gurudev came around with a microphone and asked if anyone had anything to share. I spoke into the microphone and said that I had just experienced the sacred heart of Jesus. Having been brought up a practicing Catholic, my image of the sacred heart was of a statue I remembered from school with thorns around a heart that was bleeding for mankind. That is not the sacred heart that I experienced in this yoga session. This sacred heart was huge; not in physical size but energetically. I felt that I was ONE with the hearts of Jesus and Mother Mary. I intuitively understood the love that Jesus had for all of mankind and the love that Mary had...still does...for all of us. This love that I experienced is not in or of the physical heart but an experience of God as love. In essence, I was experiencing myself as love, and love as God.

The throat *chakra* governs our ability to speak our truths. So many people on this path are still influenced by their "tribe" or root *chakra* energy. Even though they have opened the lower *chakras* to new experiences, they may not have the confidence to speak out about what they now have come to know as their truth. I try to be sensitive to others when I express my truth. The *yamas* and *niyamas* teach us to be truthful but not to hurt others in thought, word or deed. So, first, I walk the walk. If people are drawn to me and want to know more, then I am happy to talk the talk. You did not come by these writings by accident. You are ready to hear my truth. And truth *(satya)* is defined as "that which never changes.'

The third eye in the middle of our forehead is the next energy vortex in the *chakra* system. When the lower mind is quieted and wisdom begin to blossom, we look inward and may choose to live our life differently based on these experiences of enlightenment.

The seventh *chakra,* at the crown of the head, connects us with divinity. I see this *chakra* like a golden crown that royalty would wear. I see the points of the crown attracting divine energy from the heavens but I also see energy, *kundalini* energy rising up and out the crown of the head into the heavens. Sometimes I see this crown center opening like a powerful fountain. I see the energy shooting out the crown in white light usually, but sometimes in colors. Each *chakra* has a color associated with it and these colors resemble a rainbow from the dark red of the root energy through the orange and yellow shades into green, indigo and to the more subtle, cooling colors of violet and white.

Each *chakra* has its own vibration as well. These *chakras* vibrate to *bija* or seed syllables, the beginning sounds for all *mantras*. Imagine sitting in meditation and focusing on the root *chakra* at the base of your spine. Imagine energy radiating down your legs. The seed syllable for this *chakra* is *Lam*. I find that pronouncing it as "lum",really gets this *chakra* rotating, pulsating and opening. Moving upward, the second *chakra* is "vum" the third "rum" the fourth is "yum" the fifth is "hum" and the sixth is "Om". I remember this sequence with a sentence "Let's visit Rama's yellow house. O.K?"

The first letter of each word corresponds with the first letter of the seed *mantra*.

1. Lum...think limbs
2. Vum...think vaginal area
3. Rum...think of a burning rum drink in your stomach
4. Yum...think of something that is yummy and sweet in your heart
5. Hum...think of a humming sound coming from your throat
6. Om...think of this sound opening your third eye in the middle of your forehead

Allow the *mantra* to vibrate on your lips as your lips close and a hum emerges. Allow your mind to dwell in

the area of the body where this *chakra* resides. Picture
the *chakra* like a spinning wheel of energy radiating
power, color and sound.

THREE BODIES
AND THE FIVE SHEATHS

O NGOING study of the *chakras, kundalini, the nadis* and *shakti,* led me to a deeper understanding of the nature of the three bodies and the five sheaths. *Kosha* means sheath so all five of these parts of ourselves ends in the word *kosha.* They are the *anamaya kosha, pranamaya kosha, manomaya kosha, vignamaya kosha and anandamaya kosha.*

1. The physical body is called *annamaya kosha*, or **physical sheath,** sometimes referred to as the food sheath.
   This refers to the flesh and blood body so many of us think is who we are. I've come to experience that we are more than the flesh and blood body.

2. We are also an energy body that is called *pranamaya kosha* or **energy sheath.**
   It was this *pranamaya kosha* that I was experiencing in levitation. When I realized that I was up off the deck, my mind clicked in and said, 'this can't be happening', and I immediately returned to the deck.

3. The mind is referred to as the *manomaya kosha* **or mind sheath**. This lower mind is what makes us think to scratch an itch or cough to clear our throat.

These "sheaths" fit together like a knife fits into it's specially-made cover, or sheath. In the case of the mind, we have a higher mind and a lower mind. The lower mind is activated when we have longings. *Kleshas* (negative thought forms) attach to this *manomaya kosha*.

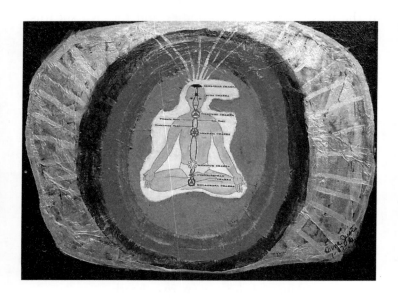

4. When we have more profound thoughts, we begin to engage the *vignamaya kosha*. This **higher mind** is what helps us understand abstract ideas. When I think, " I am not this

body…I am not this mind…I am beyond these physical manifestations". I am activating the *vignamaya kosha*. When I read the Bible, or the <u>Bhagavad Gita </u>and apply their concepts in my life, I am activating the *vignamaya kosha*.

5. The fifth sheath is called *anandamaya kosha* or the **bliss sheath**, where we experience unity. The experience of bliss is more than happiness or contentment. It is a sense of being a part of divine consciousness itself.

So let's try to understand the connection of the *koshas* to the three bodies. We do not have three physical bodies in actuality, but by combining these sheaths, we begin to understand how parts of us separate from the other parts.

A) **1st body**: *annamaya kosha* or the physical body.

B) **2nd body**: *manomaya kosha* or lower mind, the *vignamaya kosha* or higher mind and the *pranamaya kosha* or energy body. (soul consciousness)

You may have heard stories of people who have had near-death experiences. When this happens, the second body separated from the physical body. Medical staff and loved ones see a physical body present, but the person is out of body. What's "out there" is the mind, the higher mind and the prana. If *prana* leaves the body, even with life support, the person is gone. What happens to make them return? All these stories make mention of a white light, maybe a tunnel, very loving energy, beautiful music, and a blissful state.

But for some reason, the soul decides to return to the physical body. That's why this is called a near-death experience. If the person died, the first of the three bodies, the physical *annamaya kosha*, no longer has a pulse. Life force has left the body. Prana is absent. The energy body lifts out carrying with it, mind and higher mind. We know this by having experienced communicating with loved ones who have passed over. They seem to recognize us even though they have no physical eyes. They remember even though they have no physical brain.

C.) The **3rd body** is the bliss sheath or the *anandamaya kosha*. Our idea of heaven is that of a blissful place. Whatever your idea of heaven is, you probably want to go there after you leave your physical body. If it's a place, why can't we visit it now? Why do we have to wait until we die? Is that even possible? Can we live a *yogic* lifestyle and get a glimpse of heaven?

Meditation is one way to experience this bliss sheath. "Oh, I can't meditate," many people say. Many people find it difficult to meditate. They can't quiet their thoughts long enough. Don't even try to quiet your thoughts. Let them float by you like clouds in the sky. Thoughts come, thoughts go. As we develop witness consciousness, we simply observe the thoughts. They are not real, they are thought forms created to distract us from moving into a deeper state of being. Who is it that is creating these thought forms? It is our ego that wants to stay in control, that makes us think about the myriad things to think about. Allow the witness consciousness to dismiss the ego. The ego will not leave quietly. It fights for control. "But what about this," screams the ego. The silent witness watches the clouds of thought forms pass by. Witness thoughts without engaging. Become the vast blue sky, undisturbed by the storm clouds gathering. Soon, they blow away.

There are techniques for not engaging the ego. One of the most basic, that I teach in my yoga classes is to follow your breath. Breathe in and observe the breath filling your lungs...breathe out and feel the lungs collapse. Breathe in...feel your rib cage expand...breathe out...feel the rib cage contract like an accordion. Continue this pranic breathing for some time. Whenever the ego tries to distract you with thoughts, anxieties and the like, imagine them as clouds of thought forms and observe them passing by as you return awareness to the breath.

Adding a *mantra* to *pranic* breathing is effective in this regard too. Mentally repeat the *mantra* " *so hum*" with the breath. Inhale sooo until your lungs are full... exhaling humm until your lungs are emptied. *So Hum* translates as "that I am". As the higher mind ponders that thought and the *pranic* body expands with the breath, the lower mind and ego become less active. I am that breath. I am THAT which never changes. I am that I am.

There are many other *mantras* used by yogis to enhance a meditative state of being. Marrying *mantra* to *prana* is a powerful practice usually introduced to the student of meditation by a *guru*. Many yoga students use the ancient *mantra* "*Om Namah Shivaya*" as their personal *mantra*. Try it yourself and see if it resonates for you. Inhale silently chanting *Omm* pause, exhale *Namah Shivaya*. *Mantras* using the sacred names of God are often chanted as *japa* (repetition of the name of God) using *japa mala* beads. These beads are called a *mala* and are moved through the fingers as the *mantra* is repeated 108 times with reverence. For me, chanting *mantra* using *japa mala* beads is like priming the pump. After repeating the *mantra,* moving the fingers, pranic breathing, and reflection on a form of the divine engages the physical body, the mind, the higher mind, the pranic body and eventually brings us into the bliss body.

GAYATHRI MANTRA

ONE *mantra* that I learned early on the spiritual path,was the *Gayathri Mantra*. I loved the sound and vibration of this *Sanskrit* chant and would repeat it 108 times using my *japa mala* beads. While driving to and from work, I would sing the *Gayathri Mantra* at the top of my lungs. I had such love and respect for this *mantra* as a tool for bringing light to the three worlds (physical, mental and spiritual worlds)and illumining my intellect, that it became a daily devotion. Here is the *mantra*. I suggest that you search the internet to hear a *Sanskrit* rendition chanted with the correct way and try to chant it with the same intonations. Almost all *mantras* start with the *bija* syllable *om*.

Om bhur bhuvah svaha
Tat savitur vareniyam
Bhargo devasya dhimahi
Dhiyo yo nah prachodayat.

About 30 years ago, during *yoga nidra* (meditative deep relaxation) after taking a *yoga* class, I sunk into a deep reverie and in that bliss state had a vision of a beautiful goddess sitting on a lotus. She had at least five heads looking in all directions and many arms holding items. At that time in my life, I had not experienced India nor was I friends with many Indian people. I had no idea what this vision was and had no one to ask about it.

Many years later, after spending time in India, I was glancing through a book and came across a picture of the very vision I had seen in that reverie. Under the picture were the words *"Mother Gayathri."* I was shocked. I had no idea that there was a form for this *mantra.* How could that even be? I had no comprehension of the relationship between sound and light. This energy transcends the physical realm. When we grasp this, we begin to understand how a *mantra* can have a physical form. All *mantras* are associated with a specific deity... or maybe I should say that the light of the divine manifests in form when *mantra i*s chanted.

One evening, we received a phone call from my brother stating that he had heard that there had been a fatal accident near his home and that my daughter had been involved. My daughter was pregnant with her second child at the time. She had left her first born child home with her husband and was driving to the video store to return a videotape.

Upon rounding a bend in the road, a man on a motorcycle drove head on into her car. The cyclist flipped onto my daughter's windshield and was killed. At the time, my husband and I did not know the details of this event, just that she had been involved. All the way to the hospital, I chanted the *Gayathri Mantra.* We were shown into the trauma room to see my daughter lying on a stretcher with glass fragments all over her body. Her vital signs were good and there were no broken bones or head trauma. Further tests showed that the fetus was also not harmed. Did *Mother Gayathri* protect as promised?

My daughter gave birth to a healthy baby girl, whom she named Felicia, four months later. While my daughter was in labor, I was staying in a cottage by the ocean with her first born child, Monica. My family owns a cluster of cottages in a beach-side community where we spend the summer. It was just dawn and we were both in bed in separate bedrooms. As I awakened, I saw a small bright ball of light at the top of the wall where the bedroom wall met the ceiling. The orb traveled the length of the wall, turned at the corner and continued to travel around the wall. I watched it with amazement. There was no sun reflecting into the room. I have come to believe that this ball of light was the soul of the baby about to be born. Within an hour, we received word that Felicia had been born after an arduous labor with her cord wrapped around her neck. I believe *Mother Gayathri* protected this soul. My daughter and I chant regularly, and Felicia grew up chanting the *Gayathri Mantra* with us. She is now a sophomore in college. She feels that the *Gayathri Mantra* protects her when she feels frightened or alone. Last year, she had the entire *mantra* tattooed on her shoulder in *Sanskrit*. Her older sister Monica, a senior in college, has an *Om* symbol tattoo. The light of the divine manifests in form when *mantra* is chanted.

PUJA - RITUAL

CONDUCTING *puja* is an invitation to the selected deity to come for a visit. In the Hindu tradition, this ritual is done very systematically. But I would like to share the symbolism of the ritual so that if you feel so inclined, you too, can offer *puja*.

First, find a quiet place in your home to set up as a sacred place. This would be like a symbolic guest room for your spiritual guest. If we knew that God was coming to our house, we would want to clean it as best we could, put a nice cloth on the table and make preparations for the arrival. That includes preparing yourself with a bath and clean clothes. Now, send out the invitation. Call out the name of your chosen deity and invite him or her to visit you. You may do this in prayer or *mantra* repetition until you feel the presence of your beloved God in the temple of your heart. If you have an image, symbol or statue of your beloved God. You may place it on the table or altar for focus. When an honored guest arrives, we offer it the opportunity to refresh. We may offer a bath or wash up. We offer a refreshing drink of water. We may put fresh flowers in the room or burn incense. Our honored guest may be hungry, so we offer food. This ritual is in preparation for having a nice visit with your divine guest. Feel free to have a conversation with your

God as if he/she were your dearest friend. You can say anything you want and ask for anything you want. Your relationship with your chosen deity should be intimate and loving. The following is a translation of a Hindu devotional invocation:

"You are my Mother; You are my Father' You are my dearest friend; You are my nearest kin; You are my wisdom; You are my treasure; You are my Everything; You are my Lord, my loving Lord."

Give thanks and show gratitude for all that has been bestowed upon you.

Going to church for Sunday mass is a ritual that should involve preparation and dedication. I can remember going to confession on Saturday, taking a bath and washing my hair Saturday night to be pure and ready to receive the Lord Jesus in the form of Holy Communion. But how many Christians go to church on Sunday just because it is expected of them?

One of the things that can catch you up about *puja* is the ritual itself. You know how it is when we go to church and see people just going through the motions? Sometimes, *puja* can become rote. Here's a cute story to illustrate what I mean.

There was a monastery of monks who met together every morning at dawn to offer *puja* and meditate. Every morning, the ashram cat would also gather with the monks and poke around the altar, snuggling up to the warmth of the flame and sniffing the offerings. The head monk decided that the cat had to be removed to keep the monks from distraction, and ordered the cat to be tied up to a chair on the side of the altar. This went on for years. Monks came and went and the ritual remained the same. One morning at dawn, a young monk ran to the head monk crying and lamenting, "we cannot do *puja* today." When asked why not, the monk said 'the cat has died."

The head monk showed sympathy for the passing of the ashram pet, but didn't understand why *puja* could not go on as usual. "But we have no cat to tie up," was the response from the young monk.

The lesson in this story is to remember *what* you are doing and *why* you are doing it. *Ritual* must give birth to wisdom.

SOUND

ONE of the things that I loved about the Catholic Church was the sense experiences. I loved the smells, the sights, and the sounds of the mass. I sang in the church choir and enjoyed the sound that our young voices generated. I remember too, listening to the beautiful melodious sound of the boys choir in the cathedral in Cologne Germany. Those voices filled the farthest hidden nook of that beautiful Gothic cathedral. Its resonance transports listeners into a deep,still calmness within the soul and seems to call us home.

As years passed, I moved away from the ritual of the mass and became drawn to chanting. The notes of the scale seem to resonate with my body and open me up to Holy Spirit. Another technique that I absolutely love is the chanting of *mantra* referred to as *kirtan*. In this technique, a leader sings a line or phrase, and a group responds by repeating that line or phrase. The *prana* moves like bellows and the room becomes filled with movement of *prana* and *mantra*. Imagine me taking a deep breath and singing *Hari Rama, Hari Rama, Rama Rama, and Hari Hari* while you breathe in. Then while I breathe in, you repeat what you just heard with the same sequence of notes and rhythm. I sing *Hari Krishna Hari Krishna, Krishna Krishna Hari Hari* while you breathe in…then you chant it back to me. We continue singing the same chant for several minutes using bells, tambourine, drums, and harmonium, and just lose ourselves in the repetition of *mantra* and the sound of the instruments. I experience amazingly deep states of consciousness by chanting *kirtan*. What does that feel like? My experience is of energy running through my body like electricity. My whole body hums with it. My head hums with it. I sit in perfect stillness just experiencing the sensation of it. The traffic on the street hums *omm*. My hands vibrate with it. The energy inside and the energy outside of me are the same buzzing energy of divinity.

The entire universe pulses with vibration. The planets make sound even in deep space. *Mantra* and chanting seem to create a celestial sound. One year during *Maha Shivarathri* (a holy night of fasting and prayer,) I was sitting in the temple with others, chanting *"Om Hreem Nama Shivaya"* over and over. With each *mantra*, we would drop grains of rice on a paper plate. After about an hour of chanting, all of the plates of rice were poured over a *Shiva Lingam*. (an egg shaped stone revered as a symbol of *Shiva*. That year I was welcomed to bring in my own *Shiva Lingam* for the evening's service. My intention was to charge it with the spiritual energy through the chanting, that would radiate the spiritual energy of the ritual from the *lingam* in my home all year. At the end of the *puja,* after countless repetitions of the *mantra* being chanted by about a dozen people, the temple grew very quiet. In that quiet, I heard a high-pitched ringing. It sounded like a singing bowl when the rim is rubbed. I looked at my friend and meditation teacher Rajam.

"Do you hear that?" I asked in a whisper. So, what's this music?" He answered back "I hear it." with a look of wonder. No one else in that group heard the sound of the spheres but the two of us. Hearing that sound was a gift of spirit.

Another experience of a very strange nature happened after I had been hospitalized for an allergic reaction to a sulpha drug. Once the dangerous swelling had gone down, I was released home with a puffy face and itchy skin. The itching was unbearable. I was directed in meditation to make a *puja* (spiritual ritual) with water and *vhibuthi* (sacred ash), which I did. I bathed my face and scalp in the water and chanted *mantras*. This ritual helped ease the itching but I looked pretty funny with this ash drying on my face and hair. As I came out of meditation, I heard music. This was regular music played on earthly instruments. I started looking around the house for the source of this music. Nothing was playing, anywhere. I went out on the deck to see if it was coming from outside or from a boat on the river. The sound of music continued but no source was evident. For hours, after I showered and dressed, the music was a constant. In my altered state, I was listening at wall outlets. The music was everywhere. On the way to the drugstore, to pick up a prescription, the music continued. My husband returned from work and heard nothing. That night in meditation, I asked…'so, what's this music?" And the response was

"I have sent *Krishna* and his flute to distract you."

I was hesitant to include this episode because I sound crazy. Sometimes I think there is a very fine line between this spiritual stuff and lunacy. But my spiritual teachers have counseled me to just accept whatever comes, as a gift. Experiences in meditation are beyond this realm.

Many teachers on the yogic path warn about the development of *siddhis* or occult powers that manifest when we activate more subtle levels of awareness. Don't be distracted by these things. They may come and go, but stay on your path and realize your divine self. Don't get caught up in ego. Here is an example of one that happened to me.

One evening, I was sitting in lotus pose on my bed meditating. I had placed a lit oil lamp on my bureau several feet away from the foot of my bed. I like to gaze at the flame before going into deeper levels of meditation. I felt the familiar "warm fuzzies" that I had come to recognize as moving deeper. Squinting at the flame, I realized that the oil had run out and the flame had died. "Oh no," I thought. "I can't get up now. I'm sitting for meditation." I focused my energy on igniting a flame and breathed into the lamp. I never left my seated posture, several feet from the lamp. After a few pranic breaths, the flame ignited brightly. There was NO OIL in the lamp.

The ego mind would say "WOW, what a powerful yogi I am. The powers we possess are beyond our understanding. It was no more "me" who lit that lamp than "me" who was levitating on the deck. At this point, the yogi realizes that this "me" is "I" the same "I" as in I AM THAT. Jesus taught that he was a servant of the Lord, at first. Then, he said that he was the Son of God. Soon he was preaching "I and MY Father are ONE."

Because we are ONE, we can focus and tap into that divine oneness and bring into materialization what we intend, like lighting a flame in a lamp with no oil.

This is *sankalpa*,or spiritual resolution. To make a *sankalpa*, going into a meditative state and opening to divine consciousness is ideal. We don't want our egos to interfere with the purity of intent. This resolution is a promise to highest self in the form of a statement. The statement can be something along the lines of:

" I hereby resolve to life a healthy lifestyle," or whatever it is that is next for you to move forward on your spiritual path. Usually, around the new year I introduce the concept of *sankalpa* or divine resolution in my yoga classes. I lead the group in *yoga nidra* then, make a resolution for the new year.

In the year 2000, I made a resolution or *sankalpa* that I used for many years. That resolution is:

"I release all barriers to realizing my divinity."

From that date on, letting go of forms and dogma, I have allowed the barriers to fall, one by one.

What is the next step for you? If you are practicing the *yamas and niyamas* and the other limbs of yoga, take a good look at the barriers that you still have that keep you from fully merging in divine consciousness.

The Wisdom of Jnana

In 1998, on a visit to the ashram of Sathya Sai Baba, I was able to participate in a most profound interview with Baba's interpreter Anil Kumar. The following questions were presented, and Baba's responses set me up with the impetus to pursue the inquisitive nature of a jnani.

Q: What is wisdom or *jnana*?
A: It is that which makes you experience the divinity within you, above you, around you, below you. *Jnana* is awareness of God.

Q: What is the use of this j*nana*?
A: This knowledge helps you realize the purpose of life.

Q: What IS the purpose of life?
A: It's why a sick man takes medicine, so to get well and not fall sick again. This wisdom is to help you not have to be born again.

Liberation- end of the *karmic* cycle
Not to be born again is the purpose of life.

Q: Is there a connection between knowledge and liberation?
A: Here is the bulb...there is the switch, LOVE is that which connects.

Q: Do I have love?

A: You don't have love, you have attachments, friendships, possessive instinct.

Q: What IS love, then? What is that love that establishes that connection of knowledge and mortality?
A: Split of love = worldly, family love of attachment
Spirit of love = eternal, total, holistic DIVINE.

Q: Is it possible to acquire this?
A: Yes, if you have self-confidence, you can have ALL.
It is the confidence in the *"self"* the divinity within you. The *real* "I" not your skills, knowledge or ability.

Q: How do I develop self-confidence?
A: Self-confidence comes out of discrimination.

Q: What is discrimination?
A: Separating all that which is not self- *Atma* from *Anatma.*

I realize that these are very deep and profound lessons. Sai Baba says "read a little, then *experience* it." So, know yourself. He says that God's grace is necessary.

Q: What is God's grace, and once we have it, will it stay?

A: Once grace comes to you as EXPERIENCE, it
can never be forgotten.

He then gave the example of milk being churned into
butter. Butter emerges from the milk...is the product of
the churning...but will never get dissolved into the milk.
Similarly, this experience is like butter. It will never get
mixed with the old life again. And so it was with me. Sai
Baba brought me along a three fold path of devotion,
service and knowledge while living at his ashram and
while living as a householder, working a full time job
and bringing up my family. There were times when this
was a very difficult process to undergo.

There is a story of two mice sitting on the lip of
the butter vat enjoying the sweet cream. Desiring more,
they leaned in further and fell into the vat. Treading their
little legs in the cream, the mice grew tired and discour-
aged. "We'll never get out of here," cried one of the mice.
" I give up." and he died belly up in the vat.

The other mouse continued to pump his little legs
faster and faster. The cream hardened into butter, and
the confident mouse climbed out.

I have experienced the grace and the miracle of
transformation. My years at the ashram helped purify
my thoughts, words and deeds. The grace showered upon
me in the form of experience awakened the wisdom to
know myself.

The JNANIS

This new and improved life as a *jnani* was wonderful, but rather lonely. Even my spiritual husband was not into realizing the divine within. He was much more comfortable doing his meditations in front of his altar in his *puja* room, having divine conversations with his guru.

I, on the other hand, had decided to retire from teaching the duality of Hinduism, even to the children in Hindu Sunday school, and practice the non-duality of *Vedanta*. I no longer felt that God was "out there" somewhere, Divinity was everywhere. Above me, below me, around me and in me. I had experienced this and could never forget it. The rituals of the *bhakti* path, the warm connection to others by serving on the *karmic* path were lovely, but not necessary for me to realize divinity. But what I missed on this path of *jnana*, was *satsang*. (the community of like-minded souls.) I had no one to talk to about this. Thus, I put out into the universe, the need for good company. Soon, I was conducting study groups in my parlor. For the last five years or so, students from my yoga classes and other friends have been meeting to read and discuss books of a spiritual nature. The size of the group ranges from five women to fifteen women depending on the book and the interest that it generates. I refer to these women as the *jnanis*. We read, discuss and ponder how to reflect these profound teachings in our day-to-day lives. We are not a group of seasoned *yogis* either. Recently, younger women have shown interest in such topics as *karma* and *reincarnation* and are attending the *Jnani* Book Group weekly. I never know who will show up, and whoever does come, usually shares a spiritual lesson that has meaning for us all.

I have seen such amazing spiritual progress in myself and in the members of the group. We churn the milk through spiritual study and what emerges is pure, sweet butter.

Two Birds

There is a story that my friend Malaji told in our *jnani* group of the two birds in the tree. One bird sits on the lower branch chirping away and flitting from branch to branch, very taken with the ongoing activities around her. Up above, on a top branch, sits another bird very still and observant. The lower bird glanced up with envy. "Oh why can't I be like her...so quiet and self-possessed."

The upper bird answered her with:

" Oh, but you *are* me. Come up here and get away from all that chatter."

With intent and a flap of her wings, the bird on the lower branch flew up to the top branch and merged with her higher self.

So the *jnani* ladies read and discuss and churn the butter only to be reflected back to ourselves. We often end our meetings with a deep meditation session. So is there a connection between knowledge and liberation? Love is that connection.

THE FOUR PLANES OF EXISTENCE

Y OGA philosophy teaches that there are four planes of consciousness.

a. The *physical plane* is the material world. We are born, we do actions, have reactions, create *karmas,* experience pain and sorrow, and eventually, we die. Life on this physical plane is kind of like riding on a train. We get on the train move along a horizontal line and eventually reach our destination in life. We have free will and can get off at whatever station we want, but we can only move forward. We are pretty limited, or at least we think we are. We get on the train carrying our baggage and that baggage travels along with us.

b. The second plane of consciousness is the *astral plane*. Imagine getting on a sailboat. You can move along your destined path but you can tack out and tack in. You don't have to follow the train track. As a matter of fact, those souls on the train may not even be able to see you if you tack out into the ocean beyond their vision.

The astral plane is both the mind and the body.
When we think deeply and question the belief
systems that we were brought up in, we can tack
away from the norm. We can see and experience
things from another perspective.

Years ago, I took a weekend program with
Shirley McLain in NYC. It was back in her
"kooky" years and I was right there with her.
We did some amazing things that weekend.
We experienced deep meditation and did some
astral travel. On the last morning, in my meditation, I traveled in the astral realm, following the
railroad tracks to CT and the CT River to my
house in Middle Haddam. Once at my house,
I checked on the kids by slipping right through
the glass door. I didn't even have to open it. I
"saw" my son and our exchange student playing
basketball out front. Then I went looking for
my husband. I "found" him on the golf course.
Wanting to let him know that I was there, I
conjured up a white tornado., like Mr. Clean in
those old commercials.

I spun the tornado up and down his body several times then I returned to the voice of Shirley
McLain beckoning me back to that hotel ball-
room in NYC. It was time to depart for home. A
few hours later, I was back home. My husband
returned from the golf club in brown pants and
a blue golf shirt. "Oh honey, I thought I saw
you in my meditation today in your black pants
and a red golf shirt" I said.

"But I did wear black pants and a red shirt. I showered and changed at the club after playing 18 holes of golf." Chuck went on to tell me that he had played a great game of golf

"I was doing really poorly the first few holes then I don't know what came over me. I had a great score and I hit a hole in one."

" I came over you!" I yelled.
"I sent you a white tornado!"

c. The third plane of consciousness is the *causal plane*. Think of this as getting on a jet plane. You follow your destiny but there are no limitations on how you get there. You can go in a linear direction, up, down or sideways. The causal plane. Is that like cause and effect? you may ponder. I'm not exactly sure how this cosmic mind works, but it does work. You've probably read <u>The Secret</u> and know that we can make things happen in our lives with a focused mind. In the causal plane, we can put things out there and they manifest. A couple of years ago, my women's jnani group made vision boards. We each cut out pictures from magazines and visually mad representations of what we wanted to create in our lives. Our son's girlfriend Erin, cut out little pictures of weddings, a house and a happy family. She put it out there with such intent that she manifested it all. Chuck and I were concerned that our son might never get married. Now they are a happily married couple with a lovely old home that they are renovating and are expecting a baby.

Miraculous healings happen on this causal plane. I was suffering from a degenerative knee condition. The pain was so bad, we moved into a ranch- style, one level home because it was too painful for me to climb stairs. I was going to physical therapy several times a week to no avail. Chuck and I took a trip to Croatia with a side trip to Medjugorje in Bosnia. This is a very well known pilgrimage location where the Blessed Mother of Jesus has been appearing every day for years. We went to mass and to the hill location where Mother Mary first appeared. I struggled climbing the hill and had no expectations for anything. I offered prayers for others, and then on second thought, asked for a healing for my knees.

When we got back to our hotel in Croatia, I went down to the ocean to take photos of the magnificent sunset. Climbing up the stairs, I realized that I had no pain in my knees. NONE. All gone. I was healed! That was about five years ago. I have had no pain since.

This "cosmic mind" is pretty powerful. It is divine energy working through nature. I don't pretend to know exactly how it works, but I've seen enough spiritual healings to know that it does. Our grandson Griffin was diagnosed with stage four cancer when he was three years old.

Lots of petitions went up in the form of prayer for Griffin's healing. Talk about a miracle. Griffin is now 9 years old and cancer-free. Thank God.

d. The fourth plane of consciousness is the *spiritual plane*. If the third plane is likened to a jet, think of the fourth plane as a rocket ship. The spiritual plane is the absolute self. *This is the goal of yoga.* When we follow the 8-limbed path, our goal is God Realization, or self-realization. On the Spiritual plane, all is ONE. There is no form. We are simply divine energy. I have come to experience that all form exists within God.

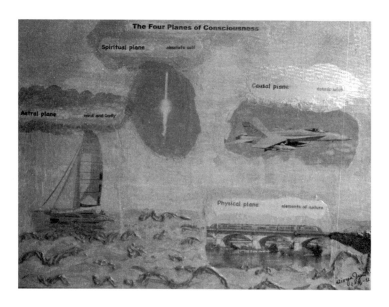

Picture that rocket ship fired up and taking off in a huge flash of light. Lots of energy is expelled to move it out of this atmosphere and into deep, space. Soon, the energy source drops away and we float through dark empty space. Imagine this deep, dark, empty space as divinity itself. Imagine every form, the planets, the stars, the Milky Way, the earth, the rocket ship all-existing within this divinity. Now, imagine the forms themselves dissolving. We are gods within God. We are ONE with God. All of us are ONE with God. When this spiritual plane is experienced, and we know that we are all one, it is very hard to harm anyone or any living thing. We experience unity. There is no separation.

Imagine a bunch of different balloons, filled with air. The air inside the balloon and the air outside the balloon is the same. It's the same air in all of the different balloons. WE are like the balloons. We may look different, come from different countries, speak different languages and worship different Gods, but if we were to pop the balloons, we would experience our oneness. We are only different in form. The absolute Self is all.

Here's another example. Imagine the absolute Self as the deep ocean. Now imagine you, your physical form as a pitcher filled with water. Imagine your pitcher immersed in the ocean. The water inside the pitcher is the same as the water outside the pitcher. Imagine the pitcher breaking. The water inside of the pitcher merges with the water outside the pitcher. The water is one. You are one with the divine.

My *guru* used to tell us that gold is ONE, jewelry is many. Imagine the many life forms on this earth as pieces of gold jewelry. There are rings, bangles, necklaces, and even toe rings. There are so many varieties. But if they all got melted down and lost their form, they would be gold.

I was at a Hindu temple with some American yoga students. One of the students asked about all of the different gods in Hinduism. Why are there so many? Who is the top God? What an interesting question. It is the same question that I asked upon entering the temple for the first time. How can Hindus worship so many Gods? The answer that I received from a learned priest was that there is no real difference among the deities. All the God forms are really one. Different people just worship a form of God that touches their heart. India is a very large country. Different states have their own language, their own traditions, and their own form of God that is worshipped at the local temple. Although forms are many, divine energy is ONE. Some devotees call God Krishna, while some prefer Rama. Some are devoted to the divine mother form of Durga. Most homes of devotees have an altar with many photos or statues of different forms of God. There is probably an elephant-headed God called Ganesha there. He represents the divine ability to remove obstacles. There may be a picture of the family guru. All are adored and recognized as forms of divinity. Have you ever seen a Hindu deity with more than one head and lots of arms? The form is representative of the almighty power of God in all forms. And so it is with the absolute self. The ultimate goal of life is to realize the self and to merge with the Divine.

This discussion reminds me of an experience that I had while meditating with my meditation teacher, Rajam Kumar, in the temple. During this time, the temple had commissioned the creation of a statue of Divine mother *Durga*. The temple had prepared a place for her and the statue was shipped from India. She lay in a large wooden crate, wrapped in sawdust and cradled as if in a casket. No one had yet laid eyes on her. During those weeks before the installation of the deity in her sanctum, I was meditating in the temple and the energy of *Durga* would come to me. Thinking that I was losing my mind, I would ask mentally, "What do you want?" She communicated to me that I was to ground her energy in this space." What? I don't know how to do that."

" You must." Was the answer. So for weeks, *Durga* energy would flow through me and I would anchor her energy in the temple. When it came time for her installation, I was asked by the women of the temple to be a part of the celebration. I wore a sari and walked around the temple holding a copper pot, filled with holy water and leaves, on my head. This procession was to honor the divine mother energy of *Durga* which was now present in the forms of all of the women present, as well as manifested in the statue that had now made her home in the temple. I had never told anyone about my experience in meditation. I didn't even tell my meditation teacher. Was it my mind? Does this divine energy need a human form to ground it? How delusional these spiritual things appear.

Another experience with my meditation teacher Rajam Kumar happened after an hour of meditation, with a whole lot of shaking going on, I felt this amazing pressure at the crown of my head. I started crying out to Rajam

"*Nataraj* is dancing on my head, *Nataraj* is dancing on my head." Nataraj is a form of Lord Shiva that is depicted as a figure dancing in a ring of fire. Logically, I know that these deities do not manifest. But maybe they do? Maybe they invite us to merge with their divine form in a way that we can understand at the time. The *kundalini* energy in my body was moving up into the crown *chakra* and in my meditative state, Lord *Nataraj* was doing the old soft shoe. Rajam settled the energy down without laying a finger on me. He chanted some *Sanskrit mantras* and swept my *aura (like a halo around the body)* with his hands. I took a few deep breaths and was "back in the body."

You might ask, "How can we merge with the Divine and live in the fourth plane of consciousness permanently, without leaving our physical bodies?" Well, I asked that question all the time. The answer that was revealed to me is that **love is** the way. When I was a teenager in love, I'd often see a pink color all around me when I kissed my boyfriend. Very sweet experience for sure as pink is the color of innocent love. Little did I know that my heart *chakra* was opening and I was actually "experiencing" puppy love. As the years went by and I married my soul mate, our sexual union brought us together in a powerful way, all of our *chakras* were in alignment. In our love and mutual respect, our bodies were joined and our energies co-mingled. During these experiences, I would often see colors, brilliant colors that would change and spiral around like smoke. This physical merging was in fact, a spiritual merging. The colors were emanating from our energetic bodies via the *chakras*. We experience and radiate love.

LOVE IS THE WAY

LOVE? Well that's easy." I love everybody," you say. Really? Do you really? Do you love that guy who cut you off on the highway today? Do you love that pedophile you read about in the paper this morning? If love is the way, then how can we cultivate love in our lives? I mean real, unconditional love. Most of us have experienced romantic love, and maternal love, even brotherly love, but unconditional love? How can we cultivate love in our *karmic* garden? Well, we start by planting seeds of love, cultivating seeds of love, watering them, removing the weeds of desire and attachment. My husband sings a song with the words "You've got to give yourself to Love, if Love is what you're after. Open up your heart to tears and laughter and give yourself to love." How can I open my heart to love? I know it's scary. We don't want to be rejected or hurt. There is even a song that says, "love hurts." But if love is the way, the only way to realize our unity, is to live in love. We can start by imagining that we are radiating "pink love energy" from our heart centers to family, friend, acquaintances, fellow workers, strangers, nations, the world!

Am I living yoga yet? Almost. Is my heart open yet. Unconditionally? Or am I still judging actions as bad. Let's now look at the different paths to yoga or union with Divine Consciousness.

THE PATH OF
SELFLESS SERVICE

THIS path of life is one of the ways to open the heart. *Seva* is the Sanskrit word for selfless service. Start the process of opening your heart by serving others with no expectation of reward. Have you ever served food at a soup kitchen? Or delivered a hot meal to a homeless shelter or to an elderly shut in? These are simple ways of beginning the process of selfless service. Observe how you feel when you serve with an open heart and non-judgmental mind. You'll feel amazingly good. Soon, as you continue seva, you will see no difference between you and those you serve. We become different colored balloons filled with the same air, different pieces of jewelry made from the same gold, different pitchers filled with the same water. Seva helps us experience our oneness. It opens our heart. This is called karma *yoga*.

THE PATH OF DEVOTION

BUT maybe you are a more devotional type personality. Maybe serving at a soup kitchen or homeless
shelter is not for you. Perhaps repeating a *mantra*, or
singing devotional songs, doing meditation or prayer is
more suited to you. Meditation can take any form on
this path from the simple deep relaxation of *yoga nidra*
(deep yogic sleep) or a guided meditation through the
chakras. Our goal is to focus on opening the heart to
experience and radiating love. This path to opening the
heart is called *bhakti yoga*. One devotional song I like
to sing is:

Love, love, love,
Love is God.
Live, live, live,
Live in love.
Expand your heart to encompass all.
Live, live in God.
Expansion is your heart,
Your heart, where God resides
God is in you, with you above you around you,
And inside you.
Live, live in love.

THE LIGHT MEDITATION

THERE is a very lovely guided meditation taught by my guru. It is referred to as the Light Meditation. I have taught this meditation to children as young as 5 years old when I taught at Hindu Sunday School. Here's how it goes:

Light a candle or an oil lamp and sit comfortably with your back erect. Stare at the flame until your eyes water, and feel like they want to close. Squint at the flame. Imagine the little beams of light emanating from the flame as little beams of divine light. When you feel ready, close your eyes and allow the image of the flame to appear behind your closed eyelids. This may take a bit more relaxing, but you'll see something. Maybe a red dot or a yellow flame…maybe the whole candlestick with a light at the top. Continue to focus on this image of the flame in your mind's eye. Imagine bringing this light into your body and down into your heart. Let the light expand in your heart *chakra* opening like the petals of a flower. Picture the light moving down your arms and into your hands. Now move the light down your body and into your legs, then bring it back up into your heart. Imagine your entire body as a body of light. As you exhale, breathe out this loving energy through your heart. You may direct this loving energy to a person or a place. Send your love and compassion to whoever may need it. Fill your town, your state, and your country, with this love light. Send it to troubled spots in the world, and out into the universe. *Loka samasta, sukino bhavantu* (May all the beings in all the worlds have happiness and peace). *Shanti, shanti, shantihi* (peace, peace, peace).

About 15 years ago, when I was president of our local Sai Baba Center, I was sitting and singing *bhajans* (devotional songs) on *Maha Sivarathri* (an auspicious night of fasting and worship devoted to Lord *Shiva)* when the words came to me "YOU are *JYOTI."* These words were the words of my *guru* Sai Baba. I pondered these words all night. "Are you saying that I am the light, Baba?" I asked. "You are *Jyoti*" was the response. Baba never gave spiritual names to his devotees, but I felt that he was calling me the light and that I should call myself *Jyoti.* This did not happen because no one else felt that this was real. I remained Patty to all who knew me, and it was Patty who responded. About five years later, Swamini Lalitananda gave me an initiation and a naming ceremony that honored Sai Baba and me by giving me a spiritual name, *"Divya Jyoti." Divya Jyoti* means divine light. When people call me *Divya Jyoti*, it is *Divya Jyoti* who responds to them. They get the highest and brightest. We all have different names and we wear different hats depending on the dharmic role we are playing. To my husband, I am Patty. To my kids I'm Mom. To my grandchildren I'm Nonnie. To those who come to me for the highest teachings, I am *Divya Jyoti.*

THE *JNANI*
OR WISDOM PATH

APERSON who is more philosophical by nature, may gain a great deal by reading scripture or having discussions about these deeper aspects of self. I am one of those people. I question everything. As a result of this inquiring nature, I gain a lot of satisfaction from sitting and listening to discourses given by swamis and learned sages.

I have been blessed beyond measure to study with some of the greatest spiritual masters of our time. Yogi Amrit DeSai, Yogi Bhajan, Sant Keshevides, Yogi Hari, Swami Jyotirmayananda, Swami Dayananda, Swami Lalitananda and of course many years of study at the feet of our beloved Sri Sathya Sai Baba. Whenever a swami would come to our Hindu Temple in Middletown, I'd be there to ask for an explanation of some scripture or story. As a western woman with such a quest for knowledge, I was received and humored. But I also was respected and taught. This path is called *jnana yoga* or the path of wisdom. I have been holding sessions in my home with like-minded people to discuss philosophy and *vichara* (spiritual inquiry). We call ourselves the *Jnanis*. Women come and women go in this group depending on their interest in the book that we are currently studying. There is never a charge for attending this group and I never know who will be there. But every week is a profound experience with wonderful women who have become my spiritual echo. We hold the mirror up to each other reflecting our divine selves to ourselves.

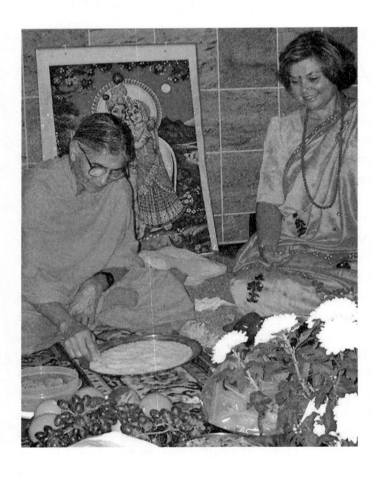

Are we living our *yoga* yet? Yoga is defined as the union of mind, body and spirit. Are we experiencing unity?

All three paths of yoga, service,(Karma) devotion,(bhakti,) and study, (jnana) Work, worship, wisdom is another way to remember these paths that bring us to union with the divine. As you walk your path and practice what you preach, talk the talk and walk the walk, you will reach your goal. Remember what Sathya Sai Baba said about the connection between knowledge and liberation. Here is the bulb...there is the switch... love is that which connects,

Love is the way,
Love, love, love is the only way.
Love is the road,
Love, love, love is the golden road.
Follow the road,
Love, love, love is the golden road.
Step by step you walk toward the lord,
Step by step, you walk toward the lord,
Step by step, you'll reach the light.

GURU—WHO IS THE *GURU*? DO WE NEED A *GURU*?

THE word *guru* roughly translates as "remover of darkness."

A *guru* is a teacher who brings us from the darkness of ignorance to the light of knowledge. In most instances, the word is used in reference to a spiritual teacher. Do we really need to find a spiritual teacher, or can we move forward with God Realization on our own? During my many years along this path, I have had many *gurus*. From that very first yoga class in the basement of the church in Old Saybrook, individuals with more experience in spiritual matters have shared their wisdom with me.

When we start the first grade, we need to learn the basics. But once we learn to read, we are restless in the first grade and ready to move on to a more challenging class. It has been said that "when the student is ready, the teacher will appear." I believe this to be true. We put the need or desire to understand something better, into the universe and soon, someone will come into your life that can help you with that concept. We all have different ways of learning. There is no "one size fits all" kind of *guru*. But truth is truth and there are a great many souls on this earth today that can serve as a positive spiritual role model. The teacher does not even need to be a living master. Many great books exist that can open your mind to new and deeper dimensions of spirit. My husband discovered his *guru,* Sathya Sai Baba in 1984 and has never wavered from that teacher. He still practices and reads Sai Baba's teachings every day. I on the other hand, have had many teachers and I have been enriched by each of them.

A *guru* is like a boat that carries us across the ocean of samsara (life's process). I had a dream once about floating in the ocean of life's process. I was the boat itself just adrift on the huge sea. The wind would take me this way and that as I experienced all that life had to offer me. I was aware that I had a goal in life, that of Self-realization, but I was adrift. In that dream, I became aware that I had a rudder. That rudder was my *guru.* It was my teacher that was helping me find the direction that would help me reach my goal. By surrendering to the teacher, rather than drifting off course, I was able to take the route that would help me to reach my destination and avoid the shoals and sandbars that might detour me.

In those days, my husband and I used to have monthly sunrise meditation sessions on our deck overlooking the river. Friends would gather in the dark and we would chant until the sun rose over the horizon. On one occasion, a friend was singing a song with words "Be the anchor of my little boat upon the sea." I opened my eyes at that moment to reflect on the sunrise and the calm water, when in the river, an orange buoy floated by, carried by the current. A boat upriver had lost this buoy just as we were singing for the protection of a teacher to keep us navigating toward our spiritual goal.

Just as we graduate from high school and go onto college, there are teachers that can teach us the basics and there are teachers qualified to teach advanced courses. Many people joke about going *"guru* shopping." I believe that it is absolutely necessary to find a teacher who not only talks the talk, but also walks the walk. We should INTEND that we raise our consciousness, and as we work at doing that through selfless service, devotion and study, if a teacher is necessary at any point, that teacher will come into our lives just when he/she is needed. Interestingly, as we follow the teachings of a respected *guru*, we also become a *guru* to others by sharing our growth with others and witnessing that growth in our lives. That is what I hope to share with this little book. Live your yoga. Read, study, practice and live the teachings of the great masters. When people ask you about your life, share with them who you are and what you have learned on this path. Encourage people along the path. Lead by example as Amma does.

Mata Amritanandamayi Devi is a great saint from Kerala, India. She states that "Motherhood, in it's ultimate sense, has nothing to do with bearing a child, but with love, compassion and selflessless. It lies in totally giving to others." If we look at Amma's life, this is what we see. Allow me to share an experience from a retreat with Amma from my journal:

July14, 2000
"I'm having a really nice time here at the retreat.

Amma's love is melting my heart. I had her darshan today. She smells delicious, even after hugging hundreds of people, she is fresh and filled with love. I felt myself melt in her arms as I cried "Amma, Amma, Amma." She whispered in my ear, "daughter, daughter, daughter'," as she rocked me in her arms. The whole atmosphere here at Bryant College is lovely. The campus is beautiful. All of the retreat participants are required to do seva (selfless service) so everything runs smoothly. The food is exceptionally delicious. Tonight, we meditated outdoors with Amma, then she served us dinner. Such an example of selfless Mother serving her children. The fresh breeze blowing as I walked back to my room after meditation, felt like a caress. Mother, as Mother Nature, is showing me her beauty. This feminine energy is all around me...Kali, Lalitha, Gayathri...I am the Goddess!."

SURRENDER

I N times of trouble, it has been reassuring to practice the principle of surrender.

Surrendering to a higher power be it a *guru,* Jesus, Rama, Krishna, the Buddha or Allah, means handing the outcome over to one who serves as the rudder of our little boat, and helps us to make it through the storms of life. We are never alone. We can always cry out for help and help will show us the way. Think of it this way: you are a child lost at the mall. If you cry out "mommy," no matter how long you cry, almost every woman in the mall is a mommy., but the chances of your mommy coming are slight. But if you call out your mothers given name, she will come and find you. Never, ever give up. First of all, you are not lost. You may think that you are all alone in this world and no-one hears your cries. But if you call out the name that is sweetest to your lips, your *guru* will find you.

Grace Troy. New York

> *May 31, 1997*
> *"On Memorial Day weekend, we headed to Rus-*
> *sell Sage College in Troy N.Y. for the Sai Baba*
> *Northeast region retreat. Our daughter had*
> *shared with us that she had two tumors in her*

*breast and did not yet know if they were malig-
nant. We decided to dedicate our devotions on
her behalf all weekend. We chanted 108 Gayathri
Mantras in the Sai Baba room twice a day with
a group of devotees. During one session, Chuck
visualized Andrea in his arms with her head rest-
ing on his shoulder. He was patting her gently on
the back. Sai Baba came in his meditation and
took Andrea. He patted her, then returned her
to Chuck. During this same session, I was sitting
on my meditation cushion chanting, when I had
the sensation of my head spinning in a clockwise
motion. A rectangular window appeared in the
space over the middle of the room and a brilliant
light shown down...a searchlight... searching for
me. When the beam focused on me, it enveloped
me in an illuminating light. From the rectangular
window, "white rain" fell. It was like I was sitting in a spotlight of grace being showered with
Divine grace. This was a very personal blessing
but the Divine invoked was due to the many souls
that were chanting the Gayathri Mantra. I just
basked in the Divine grace with a smile on my
lips, in a deep meditative trance. When the chanting was over, I was aware of the large double
doors of the room opening as people silently
filed out. In my deep meditative state, I sensed
that the white rain energy shifted and started to
escape out the door. "NO, NO," I cried silently.
The energy turned around and remained in the
room, surrounding me.*

Surrender to Sai

In 2005, Chuck and I were part of a group of eighty five people from Connecticut who went to *Prasanthi Nilayam* in India prepared to sing English devotional songs that we had practiced for months. I had packed suitcases filled with items to donate to the poor in India. As fate would have it, our luggage did not arrive. Chuck and I ended up washing our white Indian clothes every night and hanging them under the overhead fan to dry for the next morning.

Ashram life is quite regimented with early morning meditation and sitting quietly among thousands in the anticipation of the *darshan* (being in the presence of a holy man or woman) of Sai Baba. We would gather together at 5:30 a.m. to walk to the *mandir* (temple area) and sit together. The gentlemen and boys in our group used a different entrance and sat on the other side of the *mandir* separated from the women to keep distractions to a minimum. After *darshan,* we left to join the men for lunch. As I approached Chuck, one of the young men fell to the ground in a grand mal seizure. Chuck ran to the small office at the *ashram* gate and asked for an ambulance as we all rushed up to the young man on the ground.

In just a few minutes, two men came running towards us carrying a stretcher. The young man was transported to the hospital by this human ambulance mobile unit followed on foot by the rest of us. After hours of attention at the general hospital in the village, we dragged ourselves back to the *ashram* in the heat of the day, for some much needed rest. Just as I had drifted off to sleep, Chuck got up, showered and was off to afternoon *darshan*. "Ohhh," I groaned. "I can't get up yet". Some time later, I was awakened by the words of an English devotional song coming through the speakers from a performance in the *mandir*:

"Surrender to Sai
Surrender to Sai
Give Him your troubles
Surrender to Sai
Sharanam, sharanam, sharanam, sharanam,
sharanam , sharanam (surrender to guru)
There's no need to fear
There's no need to cry
It's all an illusion
To live or to die
Sharanam, sharanam, sharanam, sharanam,
sharanam, sharanam
You need not control
Don't hold on so tight
Your mind will be peaceful
as you walk to the light
Sharanam, sharanam sharanam, sharanam,
sharanam, sharanam
Have faith in the lord
He knows the design

Your heart will be lighter and
Your being divine
Sharanam, sharanam, sharanam, sharanam,
sharanam, sharanam."

"They're singing my song," I realized as I sat up on my cot. "That's my song! I wrote that song!"

Then it dawned on me that our group was performing in front of Sai Baba and singing my song without me!

I grabbed my USA scarf and ran down three flights of stairs to be met by our *seva dal* "volunteer" who acted as guardian to those of us who stayed in this apartment building.

"Luggage has arrived madam…luggage."

And there behind him were three scrawny, barefoot men with luggage on their heads.

"No, not now," I cried as I darted out the door.

"Yes Madam, NOW!" said the *Seva Dal* emphatically.

"But they're singing my song…that's my group singing for Baba! " I wailed.

"Luggage first, Madam," he said. I ran up the stairs, totally out of breath and close to tears, followed by the bearers carrying my luggage on their heads.

In the doorway, with my tons of luggage at their feet, the men stood with their hands out, waiting for a tip.

"I have no *rupees,*" I said. "No money to give."

The men stood patiently. The search went on. I found some small notes that we had for meals and thrust it into their waiting hands, bowed to them with folded palms and literally flew back down the stairs and across the *ashram* grounds toward the *mandir.* Our group was still singing, and the harmonies of the children's voices sounded like a choir of angels. I slowed my pace and listened. "What a blessing to be able to hear these songs piped through not only this ashram, but the whole village of *Puttaparthi*," I thought.

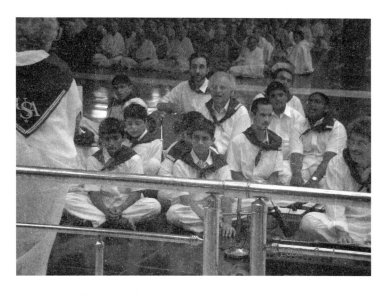

Sai Baba watched me as I crept across the huge expanse of the *mandir*(auditorium). His eyes never left me until I was seated right in front of Him and thousands of devotees and singing with our group.

This story is a good one to show how the Guru cares for His own. Baba awakened me from my sleep precisely when the song that I wrote was being sung and beckoned me to join the group in the temple area. The luggage symbolized all the unnecessary emotional stuff I was carrying around with me. I am not on the train any more.

I can leave the baggage behind. I am that rocket ship taking off in a flash of light, led by light, into the light.

The Name

There is power and vibration in a name. Remember the story earlier in these pages about the child who got separated from his mother at the mall. What a scary situation for a child. The child starts to cry "mommy" and draws the attention of many mommies in the mall, but none are his mommy. He goes on crying in fear. When the security guard shows up, he asks the child " What is your Mommy's name?" When her name is given, and announced on the loud speaker, the mom finds the child.

Often, on our spiritual path, WE are the children lost at the mall. So many *gurus,* so many practices. How can we find our way with all of the distractions? How will our *guru* find us?

When I hear the name *"Ganesha,"* I think of the elephant headed deity who is considered the remover of obstacles. Different names conger up different images and emotions. When we repeat the name of a chosen entity, that energy is attracted to us. As individuals, we play different roles in our lives and sometimes those roles are given names. Fifteen years ago, Swamini Lalitananda gifted me with a new name in a beautiful naming ceremony at the Satyanarayana Temple in Middletown. Just as a new baby is given a name, her first taste of food and new clothes, Swamiji offered *puja* and whispered my name in my ear. *"Divya Jyoti"* she whispered. "Divine Light." Then she fed me honey and showered me with rice and gifts.

Many of my yoga students followed suit feeding me, offering gifts and repeating my name.

To this day, whenever I'm called *Divya, Divya Jyoti* or *Divyaji,* THAT is who responds. The vibration of that powerful Sanskrit name resonates with my soul and my highest self emerges in response. Yes, there is power in the name. Chant the name of the Lord and you will be rewarded with the highest of vibrations, that of Divinity itself.

Swamiji and I make it a practice to grant spiritual names to our students for that very reason. As yoga teachers themselves, their students will be attracted to them by the vibration of the name and they will provide the divine light to their students until the student is ready to look within and see his or her own magnificence.

SUNDAY SCHOOL

HAVING Swamini Lalitananda live with us for a while gave me an amazing opportunity for learning, and teaching spirituality. One morning at the Hindu Temple, two gentlemen from the Board of Directors of the temple, took Swamiji aside for a conversation. I watched her nod and respond to the men. The only words I could catch in the conversation were:

" Is she ready?"

The idea of a Hindu Sunday school was the brain-child of Madhu Reddy. He felt that the American born Indian population was losing their cultural identity. The request set forth was that I start a school teaching Indian spirituality with a western approach. Surprisingly enough, I was uniquely qualified for the task. I had earned a college degree in Early Childhood Education, was a certified yoga instructor and had completed a 500-hour certificate from the Atma Vidya Ashram. That was deemed significant preparation. The curriculum for this school flowed through me in a 12-hour writing marathon. Much of the material came to me from lessons that we had presented to the children in the Sai Baba Centers.

Within six months, we had a Sunday School up and running with trained teachers (parents) and an enrollment of 80 children. I was the overall coordinator and would start every Sunday with a whole group assembly including the parents. This short segment brought us all together as a community. I was able to talk to the children and the parents together, explaining the symbolism of their beautifully complex religion. It was surprising to me that many of the things taught to the children were new to the parents as well. After the general assembly, the children would go to their age-appropriate group for projects and lessons.

One lesson that stands out in my mind regarded the various forms of God in the Hindu faith and how they are really all one. I asked the children to whom do they worshipped at home.

"Who is your *"istha devata"* (one's chosen deity) I asked. The children responded with names like *"Rama,"* *"Krishna,"* *"Shiva,"* and *"Ganesha,"* deities that they worshipped in their home with their parents. With each name called out, I put a sign with that name on a different shaped vase. There are many forms of God in Hinduism. Each state in India, and even villages, had their own statues that they use as images of God. Between the temple and my home, I had collected a lot of vases. Big ones, small ones, fat ones and thin ones. I filled a large pitcher with water and explained that each vase would represent a container to hold God energy, and that the water itself, would represent God. "Here comes *Lakshmi*" I announced as I poured water into the vase thus labeled. "And *Durga,*" as I moved along the table filling each vase with the water from the pitcher. The same water is in each vase, I casually said as each diety came to life with God energy. "Now, these vases are like the statues upstairs in the temple. The statues are containers that hold God energy." Then, we poured the water from the vases back into the pitcher. Each child was given an opportunity to have some of that water to take within his/her own body. "You have that energy in you. Your body is also a container that holds God energy."

Recalling taking the communion wafer in the Catholic Church that I grew up in, this sure felt like "communion" to me. The mystery of faith revealed.

LOOK WITHIN

THERE was an old woman who was outside the front of her house looking for something. A friend came by and asked if she needed help.

"Where did you lose it," asked her friend. "In the house," was the reply. "Then why do you seek outside? Because here is where the light is," the old woman answered. This simple story tells us a lot about why people search out *gurus*. If you don't know what you don't know, then you need someone to shine the light of wisdom to show you. If you went into the dark with just a flashlight, you would only see straight ahead of you or wherever the flashlight beamed it's light. But once the sun comes out, you are able to see what was there all along. The *guru* may point the way, but the way is inward. Go in and find what you truly seek.

Another story about the search, tells about a man in search of the treasure that his father had left upon his death. This man dug up the entire property looking for that treasure. He never did find it and left the area frustrated and angry. He actually left the family home to his sister. The sister started cleaning and preparing the house as a home for herself. Removing the floorboards under the bed in the bedroom in order to repair the floor, she came across the treasure that the brother never found after months of searching.

You see, it's not out there folks. The treasure of God lies *within* us, waiting to be discovered. And all the great *gurus* of our time are pointing to it. Go within and you shall find.

NAMASTE

AS yoga teachers, many of us end our classes by placing our palms together in front of our hearts and bowing our heads wispering *"namaste."* Usually, our students manage to allow a soft *"namaste"* to be returned to us. This simple gesture is so profound as to be a complete crash course in the philosophy of yoga. *Namaste* means, "I recognize the divine light within you."

Do we really recognize the light in the students we teach? Do we recognize the light in our family members? Do we truly believe that the light of their soul is shining forth for us to see and that the light of their soul and the light of our own soul is the same? Light is the absence of darkness. Light is made up of many colors. The light of divinity is made up of various rays. Do you recognize divinity in the ray of light that emanates from your neighbor? Jesus said to love thy neighbor as thyself. Why would he say that? I guess he doesn't know what a jerk our neighbor is, right? *Namaste.* Try greeting the next person you see with hands together in prayer position and a little bow to your head. You can speak the word *"namaste'* inwardly. Try to greet the light in that other person even if their personality is surly. If you are too self-conscious to actually place your hands in prayer position, just place your right hand on your heart and lower your chin slightly. This humble gesture expresses love. Love is the language of the heart. You are greeting the heart energy of that person and they will be affected by it. YOU will be affected by it. The more you make this simple gesture with awareness, the more aware you become of our divine unity.

My dear friend Mala Singhal tells a story about an ashram. The residents of the ashram were not getting along well and the head monk was very perplexed.

"I will ask God himself, what to do," he said to the group. God's response to the pious monk was,

"Tell them I am coming there. They will not know in which form, but I will be there."

From that day on, the ashram residents got along very well. They greeted each other with folded hands at their hearts.

"Who knows, that person I greet, may be God himself." they thought. Everyone did their work in silent gratitude. Each saw God in the other.

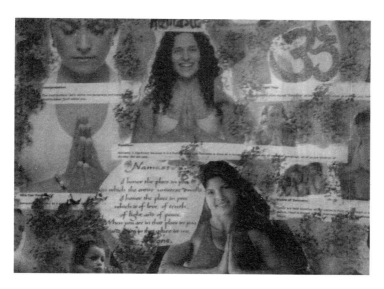

"*Namaste, namaste, namaste, namaste.*
The God in me beholds the God in you,
Namaste, namaste, namaste."

"I am one with the heart of the mother
I am one with the heart of love
I am one with the heart of the father
I am one with God."

So, if God is love, and love is God,
than Love is all there is.

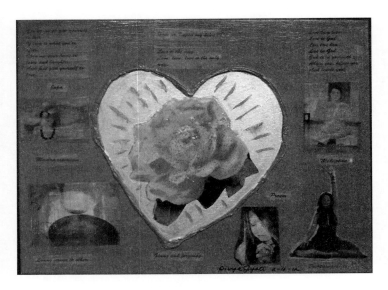

Recalling one of my favorite Beatles songs:

"Love is all there is,
Love is all there is,
Love is all there is!"

GLOSSARY

Ahimsa	non violence
Annamaya Kosha	food sheath
Anandamaya Kosha	bliss sheath
Aparigraha	non- attachment
Asana	physical posture
Ashram	monastery
Asteya	not stealing
Atma Vidya	knowledge of God
Bhakti Yoga	the path of devotion
Bramacharya	self control
Chakras	energy vortexes
Dharana	concentration
Dhyana	meditation
DivyaJyoti	divine light
Durga	divine mother
Ganesha	elephant head god
Gayathri	that which saves
Gunas	personality quality
Guru	teacher
Gurukulum	guru's school
Iswara	God
Japa	counting with beads
Jnana	wisdom
Jnanis	yogi's who study

Jnana Yoga	the path of study
Karma	activity and results
Karma Yoga	the path of service
Kleshas	negative thoughts
Koshas	sheaths
Krishna	incarnation of God
Kundalini	serpent-like energy
Maha Shivaya	holy night of Shiva
Manomaya Kosha	mind sheath
Mantra	repeating a name
Maya	illusion
Namaste	honoring god within
Nataraj	dancing Shiva
Niyamas	observances
Om	sacred sound
Patanjali	organizer of yoga
Pranamaya Kosha	energy sheath
Pranayama	breath control
Pratyahara	sense control
Puja	ritual
Rama	incarnation of god
Rajas	action or passion
Reincarnation	rebirth
Saucha	purity
Samadhi	union with god
Sankalpa	spiritual resolve
Santosha	contentment
Sathyam	truth
Sattwa	pure
So Hum	that I am
Swadhyaya	self- study

Tamas	sloth
Tapas	austerity
Vhibuthi	sacred ash
Vignamaya Kosha	intellect sheath
Yamas	abstentions

"Living Yoga" is a book based on yoga philosophy as handed down by the great sages and yogis of India. Divya Jyoti shares with us how to apply these principles in daily life through stories and personal experiences. Charming and sincere, this yogi is not only talking the talk, but also walking the walk.

Divya Jyoti DiFazio has been living a yogic lifestyle since the 1970's . Her experiences with many of the great yogis, swamis and masters of India, have highly influenced her life. As a teacher, these life experiences color philosophical lessons with a tapestry of design and depth. Divya recognizes her gurus Sri Sathya Sai Baba and Swamini Lalitananda and offers her most humble pranams to them.

Contact Divya at Divyajoti@sbcglobal.net
www.livingyogabooks.com

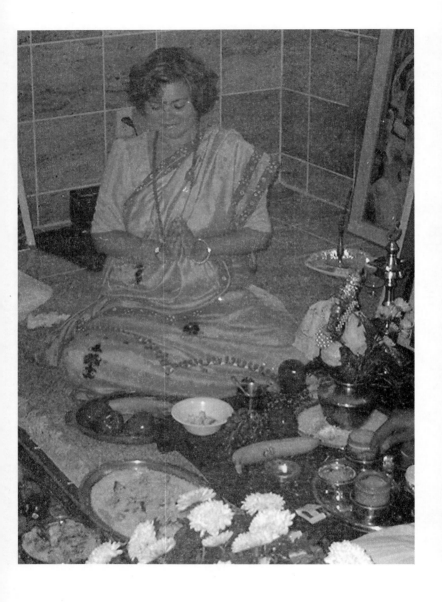